THE HEALING AND LOVE COLLECTION

Dancing with Elephants, A More Healing Way, Healing Justice

JAREM SAWATSKY

Red Canoe Press

266 Winnipeg

Winnipeg, Manitoba, R3G1X3, Canada

www.redcanoepress.com

www.jaremsawatsky.com

The Healing and Love Collection: Dancing with Elephants, A More Healing Way, Healing Justice / Jarem Sawatsky

How to Die Smiling Series -Vol. 1-3

ISBN 978-1-7753821-4-0

CONTENTS

DANCING WITH ELEPHANTS

HEALING JUSTICE

DANCING WITH ELEPHANTS

Mindfulness Training for Those Living
with Dementia, Chronic Illness or An
Aging Brain

Vol 1 - How To Die Smiling Series

Praise for Dancing With Elephants

In Dancing with Elephants, Sawatsky beautifully models a way to dance in the gale of full catastrophe, to celebrate life, to laugh with it and at himself, even in the face of personal failure and defeat.

- JON KABAT-ZINN, national bestselling author of Full Catastrophe Living

In Dancing with Elephants, Jarem Sawatsky offers a powerful example of the art of real happiness. This inspiring story reminds us just how essential it is to bring lovingkindness into every step of life, no matter how difficult the path

-SHARON SALZBERG, New York Times bestselling author of Real Happiness

... forthright and inspiring... people facing a chronic illness in themselves or in a loved one will learn from his honesty and openness.

-PETER V RABINS, co-author of The 36-Hour Day

Life can be tough and it's even tougher without the ability to find humor. You're either going to laugh or cry, so you might as well laugh. When life seems to be falling apart, Jarem Sawatsky's interesting and entertaining book reminds us that laughter is what we need to not take ourselves too seriously.

-JEN MANN, New York Times bestselling author of People I Want to Punch in the Throat

This is a beautiful and inspiring book. It is full of humor and wisdom about the pain of loss in our life, by a man who is living the severe loss of a debilitating disease. It is a book that we should all read so that loss be not transformed into anger or depression, but into love and radical acceptance.

-JEAN VANIER, national bestselling author of Becoming Human

Chapter 1 - Facing Elephants

D earest Elephant Dancer,

I know nothing about elephants nor dancing. And yet, this is a training manual and love letter for elephant dancers like yourself.

Facing elephants is something we often avoid. Most of us have elephants hidden in our closets, or hidden in plain sight. These elephants are our big, unacknowledged fears.

What are your elephants? What do you fear? Who gave you these elephants? How can you learn to love and dance with your elephants?

In this book, I serve as your guide in teaching the art of dancing with elephants. One of my big elephants is Huntington's disease—once called the dancing disease!

It's an incurable, genetic, progressive, fatal brain disease. It is kind of a combination of Parkinson's, Alzheimer's and Schizophrenia. Just picture an elephant with this combo! That picture makes me laugh now. But I have not always been laughing.

I've never really known life without Huntington's disease lurking somewhere in the corner. Huntington's is genetic and so is passed down from generation to generation. It is a slow train wreck of a disease, sometimes lasting up to 25 years from first symptoms to death. In the olden days people would say, "Stay away from those families—they go crazy as they age and it is not pretty." When I was a child, my grandmother's generation had Huntington's, as did some of our more distant relatives. Several of them were put in asylums because not much was known about the disease. I was told to not worry because a cure would surely be found by the time I developed it, if I ever did. When I was in my teens, it was mom's generation's turn–my mother had it, as did all her siblings except for two brothers, one of whom was adopted. Huntington's seemed like a massive earthquake that left mostly rubble behind. As a teen, I was part of that rubble. When I started university, I began to focus on conflict and peace studies. I was interested in finding more healing ways to deal with injustice, harm, fear, and violence. By grace, I fell in love with Rhona Hildebrand, an elementary school music teacher. Before we were married, we had to have some careful discussions about Huntington's disease—yes, you can meet my mom but she is not well and can be quite explosive. No, I guess she doesn't treat me like a son... I told Rhona she should consider seriously whether she wanted to marry into a Huntington's disease family. I nervously awaited her response. In hindsight, I learned I had two things working in my favour: 1) She was raised by people who modeled loving through life's ups and downs and 2) I am a very good kisser and Rhona was hooked. So we got married. Rhona said we needed to include "in sickness and in health" in our vows. And so we did. After a couple of years of marriage, we moved to Virginia for a year so that I could earn a master's degree in conflict transformation. During that year, we got pregnant with identical twin girls. We moved back to Canada, where our wonderful daughters, Sara and Koila, were born. I taught conflict studies at two universities in Winnipeg. Teaching turned out to be a great fit, but I knew that if I wanted to continue to teach at the university level, I would need to get my doctorate. So I applied and got a full scholarship to the University of Hull in England. We moved there when the girls were three. It was in England that I started my research into communities that practiced healing justice. I traveled around the world, visiting Thich Nhat Hanh's Buddhist community in France; Hollow Water, an Indigenous community in Canada; and the Iona Community, a Christian community based in Scotland. These places are living examples of community life where injustices are addressed with healing and love rather than punishment, judgment, and fear. During this time, my mom died from Huntington's disease at the age of fifty-eight. We had to fly back from England for her final days and the funeral. Two years later, I completed my studies and was re-hired as Assistant Professor at Canadian Mennonite University. I published two books—one about research into restorative justice and peace-building that I had written in Virginia and the other about the three communities of healing justice that I had studied in England. My career as a teacher, researcher, and author was going very well. I got a government grant to allow me to continue travelling the world searching for communities of healing justice. The girls were in school and Rhona was back at work half time. Life was good. But we knew that because my mom had Huntington's disease, I had a 50/50 chance of getting it. My mother's main coping mechanism was to deny that she even had the disease. This left too many elephants lurking in the corners. There was a DNA blood test I could take that would tell me if I had inherited the gene for the disease. My mom could have had the test done a decade sooner than she did. While denial may have provided her some comfort, it made it profoundly diffi-cult for any of us to support her on the journey. I wanted to chart a different path. First, I applied for early promo-tion at work. Once I was approved, both me and my brother had the testing done. I was positive. He was not. I would develop the disease. My daughters now had a 50/50 chance of having the disease.

For me, the news was both shocking and not shocking at

all. I had always felt like I would get the disease. That insight provoked me to enjoy life in the present. However, having a doctor tell you that you will get this disease is, of course, different than listening to your own inner voice. The genetic counsellor had to make sure I wasn't suicidal over the news. When she asked what we were going to do next, I said, "We will throw a Movers and Shakers party with friends to welcome the next part of our journey." She asked if I was kidding. You can read about the party in Chapter 5 – Celebrate Everything.

The same day we learned my diagnosis, we told our girls and went on a short family vacation to process it. The doctors could not give me a timeframe for the onset but I started to visit a neurologist every eight months for a checkup. Four years later, in 2014, I began having symptoms. When it was time to see the neurologist again, I put together a self-assessment, comparing myself to the previous year. Rhona added to the list and we shared it with the neurologist and the social worker from the Huntington Disease Society. Here are some highlights from that list.

MOVEMENT (BODY):

- stiff ankles
- progressively poor typing skills
- involuntary foot and toe movement

- finger movement
- elbow movement, lots of spilling
- decreased spatial awareness – knocking into things
- tingling sensation in the top of head
- painful sensitivity to loud noises
- ringing in my ears
- some swallowing problems
- night-time leg twitches
- more sick days from work than ever before

COGNITIVE (MIND):

- difficulty moving to the next task at work
- inability to multitask
- very distractible, can't keep focus very long
- hard time deciding on priorities
- tend to get an idea in my head, then get fixed on it
- altered sense of time—it seems to move very slowly, and I am more impatient
- hard to remember to follow through on short, easy tasks
- overwhelmed by email, and don't open most of it
- harder time making decisions
- hard to sustain complex research exploration
- slowed mental functioning

- loss of ambition—hard to self-motivate or initiate
- hard time remembering short grocery list
- hard time remembering/accessing the word I am looking for
- tend to take on job assignments at work and then not get work done
- foggy brain

PSYCHIATRIC (EMOTIONAL AND relational)

- depression
- don't seem to feel fear in situations I used to feel fear (e.g. heights)
- hard to move out of anger
- tend to be easily irritable
- avoid social settings
- constantly feel like a failure at work
- increasingly tired in the evenings and likelier to stay home and not relate to others
- tend to care less about mistakes
- loss of spontaneity – prefer to know what is coming

Rhona and I met with the neurologist and a social worker. After a bunch of discussion, the neurologist told us that it was time for me to quit work. This was in early July. Again, we went straight on vacation—a road trip across Canada—lots of time to process our new path, again.

On the advice of friends, we added a golden lab puppy named Kobi to our family. Sara and Koila are 15 now. Kobi is two. And I am literally stumbling my way into learning about loving, letting go, and living in the present moment.

I understand the agony, pain, and struggle of having your world turned upside down by disease and aging. I have watched Huntington's move through three generations. I look into the eyes of my daughters with the full knowledge that there's a 50/50 chance that they too have Huntington's, passed on by me. After they turn 18, they will need to wrestle with whether or not to get the DNA test done. It is possible this disease may take another generation, my girls.

This is hard for all of us. In many ways, I have had lots of advantages in life. I have made studying conflict and healing my life's work. I do not want agony to be the main story of my life. I think agony, on its own, is toxic. I do not want to pass agony, fear, or violence onto Sara, Koila, or Rhona. So I have been experimenting on myself to find a healing way to face disease.

I am two years into these experiments and explorations. I will share my results with you. To help you understand the way I am trying to live well with disease, I need to first share the stories and the wisdom of some of the people who have influenced me the most on this journey.

When you find out that you are dying from an incurable disease, a kind of clarity can emerge. It is the clarity to distinguish between what matters and what does not matter. Having four university degrees and having experienced three generations of a debilitating disease, I had a lot of sorting to do. This book chronicles what I see as important. It is my cheat sheet for facing disease and aging in a healing kind of way.

When I had to "retire" at age 41 from my work as a university professor, I had hundreds of books. I gave away almost all of them. I saved the handful I thought might be helpful for me in learning the art of dancing with elephants.

The author with the greatest number in my little library is Zen Buddhist Master Thich Nhat Hanh. While he is not quoted much this book, Thay—as his students call him—lies at the heart of it. Thay is responsible for bringing a revitalized Engaged Buddhism to the west. He was nominated for a Nobel Peace Prize by Martin Luther King Jr. I had the privilege of spending time at his community, Plum Village, as part of my research on healing justice. Thay is an author of more than one hundred books. I find his writing and speaking deeply valuable. It is inspiring but also very concrete and practical. I was deeply shaped by Thay's focus on practicing wisdom in everyday life and living that wisdom in a community. In this book, I try to maintain this focus: true wisdom, lived in the everyday, supported in a community. The summer I was at Plum Village with my family, Thay taught the five mindfulness trainings. Each of the five parts of this book reflects one of these trainings.

Each section also includes an interview with a leader in the field of finding more healing ways of living. The featured teachers include the following:

Jon Kabat-Zinn, is the author of 10 books on mindfulness, trauma and health. He is known for mindfulness based stress reduction (MBSR) trainings which more than 16,000 people have successfully completed. MBSR was designed to develop relaxation and calm self-awareness, a reliable foundation for facing the "full catastrophe" of stress, pain, and illness—indeed, of life itself. In Chapter 6 Jon Kabat-Zinn dares us to focus on living now, rather than being paralyzed by the life we cannot live.

Patch Adams, M.D. who was made famous by the hit movie starring Robin Williams. Patch has been working on building a model hospital, modelled as an ecovillage where doctors and patients live together and where the doctor and the janitor get paid the same salary. Patch estimates he has been present at more than 10,000 deathbeds. In my interview with him in chapter 11, he talks about dying well and living well.

Lucy Kalanithi wrote the bestselling book *When Breath Becomes Air* with her 36-year-old neurosurgeon husband, Paul, as he was dying of stage IV metastatic lung cancer. Lucy, who is also a medical doctor and professor, spoke with me about true love in the face of diseases like cancer.

John Paul Lederach is the author of more than 22 books on conflict transformation, peace-building, and healing. John Paul—my former professor—and I discuss how his professional life and his faith has helped and hindered him in supporting his wife, Wendy, who has Parkinson's disease.

Toni Bernhard was a law professor at the University of California-Davis for 22 years until some fibromyalgia-like illnesses forced her to retire. In chapter 29, Toni and I discuss the three books she has written since, including *How to Live Well with Chronic Pain and Illness.*

The rest of the book offers glimpses of my wrestling, laughing, and stumbling my way into healing. Not the kind of healing that takes away the disease but the kind of healing that awakens the heart to love. I call this dancing with elephants because dancing is a playful way of engaging that which we fear most. Those who know me well know that playfulness is a major practice for me, as is the intentional use of humor. Suffering is real and must be faced head-on. But suffering alone is not enough. On the other side of suffering can be joy—and also more suffering. We must learn to dance with both.

Our culture offers abundant advice on how to achieve financial and career success, but there are very few books on how to embrace the downward path of losing your mind. We have success tips for leaders, but almost no "success tips" for the billions of us facing disease, dementia, and aging. This book is for those billions. Together we will explore the art of dancing with elephants.

I invite you to join me in this dance.

PART I
REVERENCE FOR LIFE

Chapter 2 - Embracing the Hard Things

On Avoiding the Hard Things

Do prayers ever piss you off? Sometimes they piss me off. In my teens and twenties, I was a wilderness guide, leading group canoe trips. Sometimes participants on these trips would pray that it wouldn't rain. Even in my teens, I knew this made no sense. Sometimes I would prod.

"Do you want the trees and animals to die? They need rain."

"No," they would say. "We just don't want it to rain on us."

"Oh, so you want it to rain on the other groups I take out this summer, but not your group?"

"No," they would say. "God can make it rain on the trees and animals but not the people."

I already realized as a teen that it requires substantial mental (and sometimes theological) gymnastics for people to be able to justify a view of the world in which uncomfortable or unpleasant things shouldn't happen.

On the Way We Ride the Wave

This fall, I returned to that same wilderness of Canadian Shield country. It felt like coming full circle. Crossing paths with my younger self, I was reminded of the wisdom I could receive only by listening to the heartbeat of the wild. The temptation to try and insulate oneself from the hard things remains both common and under-standable, but I still don't want to run from the storm. I don't want to run from the hard things. Healing is not the absence of the storm. Healing is the way we ride.

Driving alone on the prairies after going to the funeral of a young man, and thinking about my own chronic illness and about rain, I wrote this poem:

Nobody Wants the Rain
Everybody wants green scenery
Nobody wants the rain
Everybody wants food on the table
Nobody wants the rain
Everybody wants the colourful rainbow
Nobody wants the rain

Everybody wants water in their bodies
Nobody wants the rain

I went to the prairie,
The Expander of Horizons
To ask about the rain
I stood on the edge of the world
And watched the rain coming all around
And the prairie proclaimed a vision
Each time the gift of rain was offered
the people ran in fear
Heart's fear perverts darkness into evil
Missing the gift of life hidden in the cloud
Let it rain down, let it rain down
Let it rain down on me

Everybody wants green scenery
Nobody wants the rain
Everybody wants food on the table
Nobody wants the rain
Everybody wants the colourful rainbow
Nobody wants the rain
Everybody wants water in their bodies
Nobody wants the rain

I went to the mountain
The Giver of Wisdom
To ask about the rain
I knelt on ancient rocks
Fifty billion years awake

and the rocks spoke to me
The rain shapes and molds us
and turns us into sand
These rain-shaped rocks
Feed the earth as their dust becomes soil
The mighty mountains are transformed
By but a tiny drop of rain
Let it rain down, let it rain down
Let it rain down on me

Everybody wants green scenery
Nobody wants the rain
Everybody wants food on the table
Nobody wants the rain
Everybody wants the colourful rainbow
Nobody wants the rain
Everybody wants water in their bodies
Nobody wants the rain

I went to the ocean
The Alpha and Omega
To ask about the rain
I sat on the ocean's edge
As but a tiny grain of sand
And the ocean questioned me
Where is my beginning and
where is my end?
Ocean's edge is hard to find
On shore? In sky? Inside my body?
The ocean's end is its own beginning

Let it rain down, let it rain down
Let it rain down on me

We cannot learn to revere life if we cannot wrap our hearts around the idea that suffering exists. The art of dancing with elephants is not the elimination of suffering. We don't kill the elephant. We learn to dance with it. All living beings suffer. To revere life, we cannot remain in denial but must understand that suffering and death are inevitable. This truth is not the end of the story but it is a necessary starting point on this journey.

Once we become comfortable with the idea that suffering exists, we need to learn to let go of fear and replace it with love. This is the focus of the next chapter.

Chapter 3 - Replacing Fear
with Love

The next step in learning to dance with elephants is to learn to overcome fear. Fear lies at the root of much unnecessary suffering. Overcoming fear will dissolve some kinds of suffering. The suffering that remains needs to be accompanied by love.

On October 27, 2010, I tested positive for the gene for Huntington's. This meant that I would get the disease that had killed my mother and a number of her relatives. Among other things, this disease is a long, slow degeneration to death. Through this disease, over the course of about twenty years, I get to practice the spiritual discipline of letting go of everything that I had thought made me human: eating, walking, sitting still, control of muscles, speaking.

Exactly one month after testing positive for the Huntington's gene, I was to preach in the small Christian church community where I grew up. I agonized about what to say. One of the practices that was giving me joy and freedom at that time came from a meditation that I had learned in Plum Village. Fresh with the perspective that I should speak out of my experience (rather than primarily out of my thinking), I modified a meditation on bones to use language that more of my Christian friends would understand. That Sunday, I told the community about my diagnosis. I told them that if there is an elephant in the room that won't go away (like Huntington's) at least we can learn to dance with it. And I taught them the practice that was helping me learn how to dance with the elephant. It is a practice of transforming fear into joyful dancing, called Corpse Prayer. It's not an easy practice but it does seem to bear good fruit in me and others. And so I offer this practice to you as a tool that may help you begin to dance with your own elephant.

Corpse Prayer

I want you to take a moment to imagine the last three minutes of your life. Where will you be? What will you be doing? Who else is there? Will it be sudden? Will you be suffering? Will you have suffered for a long time already? What emotions and thoughts will you be experiencing?

Imagine the scene as if you were watching it on a TV screen. Notice the emotions that arise within you as you watch. Do not identify yourself with these emotions, but recognize that they are rising within you. If these emotions are primarily fear and anxiety, then you know this is a tender topic that needs your careful attention. Let us practice loving yourself at the point of your death.

As you picture yourself dying, try saying these phrases:

Be not afraid.
I give thanks to God who created all things good.
In Christ, all things hold together.
I am not entitled to life without death.
I embrace sacred life. I embrace sacred death. I embrace the growing and crumbling in between.
Smile at yourself in the silence…

Now picture the moment your body is being buried. Think of that moment when your body returns to the earth, when your coffin is lowered and reaches the end of its journey.

Picture yourself there. See the movie. Notice the emotions that arise within you. Do not identify yourself with these emotions but recognize that they are rising within you.

As you picture yourself dead and just starting to decay, try saying these phrases:

Be not afraid.
I give thanks to God who created all things good.

In Christ all things hold together.
I am not entitled to life without death.
I embrace sacred life. I embrace sacred death. I embrace
the growing and crumbling in between.
Smile at yourself...

Now picture your body two years after your death, when your body is decomposing and the worms are eating your flesh.

As you picture yourself dead and well decayed, try saying these phrases:

Be not afraid.
I give thanks to God who created all things good.
In Christ all things hold together.
I am not entitled to life without death.
I embrace sacred life. I embrace sacred death. I embrace
the growing and crumbling in between.
Smile at yourself in the silence...

Now picture your body eighty years later, when all that is left is bone, or move even further into the future and watch as even your bones turn to dust. Attend to your emotions.

As you picture yourself dead and turning to dust, try saying these phrases:

Be not afraid
I give thanks to God who created all things good

In Christ all things hold together.
I am not entitled to life without death.
I embrace sacred life. I embrace sacred death. I embrace
the growing and crumbling in between.
Smile at yourself in the silence…

For me this practice is freeing, even humourous. If in the end all is dust, I can let go of some of my fear, anxiety, and self-absorption. If in the end all is dust, then now is the time to enjoy, to play, to love. The fruits of this kind of freedom are countless.

Transforming Road Rage

Of course, life is still full of struggles. But replacing fear with love helps us as we face them. Let me give just one taste of the fruits of living with less fear.

One day last year, I was driving our car in downtown Winnipeg, heading out with my wife, Rhona, on a lunch date. From behind us, we could hear a horn blaring. Some seconds later, I stopped for a red light and saw a young man in a large, shiny truck with extended suspension in the next lane. I looked up at him. He was yelling and glaring at me. In the past, I probably would have been afraid and would have suppressed my fear until it came out later, directed at some other target. But this time, things unfolded differently. I glared back at him. As he struck different poses, I copied them. I saw his passenger window was open, so I rolled down my driver's side window. I think I wanted to hear what he was saying. But before I made any plan or intentional decision, I found myself calling out to him, *"Parlez-vous Francais?"* politely asking if he speaks French! On my right, I saw my wife instinctively pretending to be a deaf person reading an imaginary book. On the other side of me was the young man in the big truck, full of rage. After an awkward silence, he said "No," and gave a big sigh. He de-escalated and backed right down and so did I. Who knew the language of love (French, I mean) had the power to transform fear and road rage into humour. After my wife's disappearing act ended, her fear turned to laughter. "Did you just pretend to speak only French?" she asked. "Yes," I answered, though in truth I speak very little French at all.

I know this was probably not the most honest or most loving response. But responding with playfulness rather than fear transformed the situation. When you let go of fear, a new vista starts to emerge. This new vista is a meadow, with plenty of room to explore, to play, to laugh, and to love. Perhaps the Corpse Prayer can help free you. Or if that doesn't work, try laughing.

There is much healing we can do when fear is replaced by love. Fear makes us defend life, like some possession, at all costs. Love provides a way to revere life without treating it as a possession. Great elephant dancers need to start learning anew to revere life. To help us hold sacred life as it is, we need to learn the art of seeing.

Chapter 4 - Letting Go

It is only when we lose something or have it taken from us, that we realize we feel entitled to it. Then we have to wrestle with what life means without our entitlements. Anyone who has dementia, chronic illness, or an aging brain knows what this feels like.

This poem, "Letting Go," represents some of the questions I have been asking myself. I wrote this while still working and anticipating that I would need to go on long-term disability.

Letting Go
How deeply can I let go of entitlement?
Can I let go of entitlement to work?
To status
To being productive

To right livelihood
To gainful employment
To forms of vocation

Can I let go of the entitlement to body control?
To controlling movement of limbs
To controlling bladder and bowel
To looking "normal"
To eating quietly and cleanly
To a voice that is respected

Can I let go of entitlement to emotional stability?
To controlling anger
To a predictable response
To understanding my own responses

Can I let go of the entitlement to self-reliant
transportation?
To drive a car
To ride a bike
To walk long distances

Can I let go of the entitlement to be accepted by others?
To smiles from strangers
To lovemaking with my lover
To gratefulness of students
To being asked for help
Can I let go of entitlement to time?
To a future
To grandchildren

To being at a child's wedding
To memory

Some entitlements are harder to give up than others
Yet it is not our entitlements that make us human
But rather Creator's gift of a still fragile life
On the other side of entitlement lies more joy than
sorrow
How do I get to the other side?

PERHAPS POETRY CAN BE part of the art of dancing with elephants. Thich Nhat Hanh has always encouraged his students to write poems. When you write a poem, the poem lives in you.

So I dare you to write poetry. If you are not poetic, take me as your guide and write bad poetry. It does not matter if you think of your poetry as bad or good but rather that it comes from the heart and that it helps you walk in a healing way.

Ask yourself: "What do I need to let go of in order to embrace life in the here and now?"

Write a poem to teach yourself to let go of entitlements.

Then sing it in the shower. Chant it as you walk. Say your words through the tears, the fears, and even through the laughter.

I have one more dare for you. Share your poetry on letting go. Let go of your fear of what others may think of your poetry. Share it with your circle of friends and consider sharing it on my Elephant Dancers Facebook Group. As we practice our poetry and the art of letting go, we can be nourished by one another's insights. So go to this page: www.jaremsawatsky.com/facebook. Let me know which email to send your group invitation to and I will send it to you. Then you can post poems and reflections for other elephant dancers to see. Let go. I dare you.

Chapter 5 - Celebrating Everything

A Celebration for Losing Your Mind

Western culture is better at celebrating beginnings than endings. We know what to do with births and marriages but don't do as well with deaths or divorces. We know even less about celebrating what we see as disability.

When I was told I had the gene for Huntington's and that I would get the disease, the genetic counselor asked what I planned to do. I said we would throw a big party. She thought I was joking at first. But I wasn't. My Huntington's diagnosis brought immense changes to my life and my family and we needed to mark this transition. We needed to eat and laugh together, to remember and celebrate as a community.

Huntington's disease, which causes constant uncontrolled

movements, used to be known as a dancing disease. So we decided that this party should be a Movers and Shakers party. Originally, I wanted to invite everyone to bring a drink or food to share that shakes—martini, jello, milkshakes. In the end we let this piece go, but we did eat together—homemade wood-fire pizza, drinks, and lots of desserts.

If you look at almost any culture, you can see that healing and peacemaking steps are often steeped in the practice of eating together. In most cultures around the world, it would be unthinkable to try to make peace without the practice of feasting together. Sharing the very things that make for life—like food—is a sacred way to be together. For me, it was a profound time of communion.

Knowing that memory loss is a part of Huntington's disease, we were encouraged to start creating memory books—pictures and stories of where we've been. In the long-run, these would be invaluable. So as part of our party, we set out to create a book—of pictures of the party, but also of stories, emails, and memories of friends and family. We asked a professional photographer (focphotography.com) to come record the event. She took the job but refused payment! People from around the world, as well as friends at home, shared memories of me. It was as if they were holding up a mirror, reflecting back to me who I have been. What a gift!

We are surrounded by many great friends. Hearing our

news was traumatic for them. Many wanted to help but didn't know how. At this event, some of our friends reminded us that we needed to be teachers for them in how to walk this path together. People wanted to help but needed to be shown how they could be supportive. So we organized our Movers and Shakers party and invited our various circles of friends and colleagues to celebrate "my retirement" in a way that made sense to us. We needed to mark this event, which was both an ending and a beginning, with the same conviction we had marked previous life events. Had someone else planned the party, it might not have felt right for Rhona and me. We put together an epic event, a party that was a profound and healing celebration to help us and our community mark my transition to living with Huntington's disease.

We didn't set out to create sacred time. But after the party, a person who had been to the party spoke about how profound the experience was and how incredible it felt to share that party with our family and our circles of friends. In some ways this was an awkward event. We didn't have a model to follow. Would this be a time of mourning or celebration or boring speeches? It turned out that our Movers and Shakers party was a time of compassion—which literally means "to suffer together"—and celebration. I highly recommend it to anyone!

For elephant dancers, celebration is a mindfulness training. Celebrate everything. We do not know what will happen tomorrow but we can find an excuse to celebrate today.

Chapter 6 - Living the Life You've Got with Jon Kabat-Zinn

> From our perspective, no matter what diagnosis you come with or what's wrong with you, there is more right with you than wrong with you—no matter what is 'wrong with you.'

It was like someone just smacked me on the head and I fell awake. More right with me than wrong with me? The man speaking knows I have Huntington's disease. In fact, he has spent his whole career working with people who have chronic and terminal diagnoses. At his own Stress Reduction Clinic, he has helped thousands of people who are facing profound suffering.

He kept saying it throughout our conversation: "If you are not dead yet—people, as long as you are breathing, from our perspective (big smile) there is more right with you than is wrong with you, no matter what is wrong with you."

Living on long-term disability with a chronic and terminal condition, I have a huge list of specialists I can call on to help with what is wrong with me: neurologist for brain problems, psychiatrist for problems in the psyche, speech and language pathologist for speaking problems, dietitian for food problems. The medical literature on my condition divides it into stages based on the inability to do things. More negative, problem-based thinking! I need to be careful not to see myself as one huge, fragmented problem. Although the experts call themselves health professionals, it seems to me that they are forced to act as disease or problem specialists.

But Jon Kabat-Zinn was pointing toward a different, more freeing way.

Feed What Is Working Rather than What Is Not

Jon founded Mindfulness-Based Stress Reduction (MBSR), an eight-week program that is used in hundreds of hospitals around the world. His books have sold millions of copies because he is onto something. During our conversation, he explained to me the purpose of MBSR.

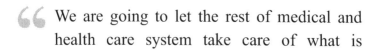 We are going to let the rest of medical and health care system take care of what is

'wrong with you' and instead we will pour energy into what is right with you, in the form of affectionate and kind attention—and we see what happens. What happens is, people are tremendously energized by that invitation.

Jon is clear that there is a role for western medicine but he is also aware that the health care system sometimes contributes to unhealth and that those with profoundly difficult, long-term conditions often fall between the cracks and gaps.

Jon's work is to dare people to live better lives, even if no cure is possible. While he draws on Buddhist approaches, he is not a Buddhist. Mindfulness, he told me, is a way to live life: "The more you cultivate this present-moment, non-reactive, non-judgmental, open-hearted presence—or attention or awareness—the more it can become your default mode."

When I am told there is no cure for my condition, it is easy to focus on "Why not?" or "Poor me" or "I don't want to die." That reaction adds suffering to suffering. I sought out Jon because I knew he could teach me about living well to the end. He told me, "We all have a terminal condition, called living. The question is, are you still living?"

There Is a Way to Hold Your Suffering and Be at Home in Your Body

66 The basic message is a very hopeful one. There is a way to hold all of your story—the full catastrophe—that is not only integrating and joyful, in a certain way, but that also gives your life back to you in ways that are very hopeful and optimistic."

Jon knows his task is to liberate people. In working with people with chronic and terminal conditions, he first focuses on freeing them from their own stories and from the stories they've absorbed from others, stories which suck the life right out of them. His approach is rooted in wisdom gleaned from witnessing thousands of people who have been in this spot and who have figured out how to get their lives back. This is hopeful. It is the hope of knowing that what you need is right here; it's not the hope of escaping from this place. I like this hope.

During our conversation, he challenged me: "Yes, maybe you have deficits or losses and they may get worse in the future, but how you are in relation to them in this moment can make an enormous difference in coping with the things that cannot be changed. We know enough about science to realize that your thoughts, emotions, and the stories you tell yourself about the future—about how inadequate you are, or how hopeless things are, or whatever— all that affect your very biology. You need to learn to be at home in your body, mind, and heart."

I commented, "Those people who are at home with themselves cause a lot less suffering to those around them and those trying to help them. The ripples keep on going."

"Yes, that is right," he said, getting excited. "This is not just a nice little stress reduction for myself to lead a happier, healthier life. When you do this kind of interior work, the social effects are profound: not just in your family (although they benefit) and not just in your workplace, but throughout the world, because of the ways in which the entire universe is interconnected."

Reclaiming the Present Moment

For Jon, the key to living in a healing way is to reclaim the present moment. Listen to some of his insights:

> *While you are still breathing, no matter how long you have to live–and that is an unknown —can you reclaim the present moment? That is tremendously healing, even in profoundly difficult situations.*
>
> *We are all finite beings. We are all going to die. But the real question is, before we die, can we live fully? The dying usually takes*

care of itself. It is the living that is the real challenge.

> *Am I living the life I am supposed to be living or am I living a caricature of that life? Am I so distracted and caught up in getting someplace else that I am missing the preciousness and the uniqueness of moments on the way to wherever it is I think I need to go to be happy?*

As one with a chronic condition, I need to be careful not to get caught in the past—in yearning for the life I had. I also need to be careful not to get caught up in the future —mourning the life I will not have. Both the past and the future can be toxic for us. When we let go of trying to get someplace else, we fully live each moment. Once we start being nourished by the present, our craving for the life we cannot have diminishes.

Losing Your Senses Without Losing Who You Really Are

"Even if you pour energy into what is right with you and you are compassionate with yourself, you will still lose yourself over time," Jon said. "As we age, we are all losing our senses, biologically. But we are not losing who we really are."

I know these are not flippant words. Jon's father had

dementia for ten years. He offered more advice. "In terms of the progression of cognitive deficits, or losing our senses—hearing, touch, taste, or whatever, or balanced walking—those losses can be folded into the meditation practice," he said. "Instead of the greatest scourge, they can become the greatest teacher of all."

This is one of the great gifts of mindfulness. You can use the very thing you fear as a tool to replace fear with love. I know he was offering me powerful medicine.

From the time I was 16 years old, I have meditated looking at my steady hands, knowing that someday they might not be steady because of Huntington's. Each time, I meditated until I was OK with this possibility. Meditating on my hands has freed me from the expectation that my life should not include having Huntington's disease. It has taught me not to get caught up in hoping for a future that may be impossible for me. It has taught me to hold my career lightly and to not over-identify with it, as it could easily end. There is a mountain of suffering that I have not had to tunnel through because I lucked into a meditation practice in my teens.

Jon was trying to save me from suffering over things that do not require suffering. This was an act of love.

Mindfulness as a Radical Act of Love

As our discussion neared its end, Jon looked at me and tried to offer a raft of compassion for the journey ahead.

He wanted to make sure I was getting the heart and spirit of his message. "When all is said and done, all that mindfulness is, is a radical act of love," he said. "To drop in on yourself in the present moment and to string some of these moments together in open-hearted presence. It is a radical act of sanity and reclaiming your humanity in the only moment any of us ever have. And that changes everything!"

If, in the end, it comes down to living in love, I think I can do that. Even with holes in my brain, I can love. Even with no cure, I can love. Do I need speech for love? Do I really need to hold my body still to be able to love? There are a lot of things I need to let go of, and I have tried to work on those, but if what's in the center is love, to me that is a liberating idea that connects me with everyone.

Jon knows choosing to face reality and to live in a healing way is not easy. "This is a deep existential choice, which is itself a radical act of love," he said. "Choosing not to fall into despair when that is a kind of default mode is hard. Some people don't make this choice. And yet this is something every single person is capable of doing. It is not like you need to go to college or be a university professor, or anything like that. Any single person is capable of doing the work of waking up, if they have the appropriate support and motivation. It means living our lives as if they really matter, and they do."

This kind of compassion or mindfulness is not about learning the right ideas or concepts. It is about practicing compassion daily, on a lifelong basis. Whatever senses we have available to us—hearing, vision, touch, smell, and taste—we can use them to wake up to non-reactive, non-judgmental, open-hearted presence—to love. All of Jon's books offer very specific ways to awaken the heart of compassion.

I recorded our interview as part of a five-part series, "A More Healing Way: Video Conversations on Disease." In the full video conversation, we explore other themes as they relate to mindfulness, such as global warming, President Trump, indigenous traditions, and full-catastrophe living. You can also hear Jon recite two of his favorite poems. To get a free copy of the video series, sign up for my Readers Group and I will send it your way.

(www.jaremsawatsky.com/more-healing)

PART II
TRUE HAPPINESS

Chapter 7 - Living Beauty Awake

When my dear friend Kathy Barkman died, her husband, Lyle, asked me to offer a teaching at her funeral. This section, with some minor alterations, is the teaching I gave at her funeral on March 29, 2016. Kathy died from cancer at age 57. She had also lived with Multiple Sclerosis for many years. Kathy was a person of deep joy and happiness through all the ups and downs of life. She is a great example of true happiness.

When Lyle asked me to offer a teaching, he said there was a new song by Steve Bell, a Juno-Award winning artist (and friend) that totally captured the essence of Kathy's stunning, simple beauty. He sent me the lyrics and a demo of the song. You can hear "Let Beauty Awake" by going to this website:

https://soundcloud.com/steve_bell/let-beauty-awake.

I listened to the song while contemplating the life and death of our dear sister and friend from my own perspective, as someone with Huntington's disease, trying to live well in the face of certain death. After listening repeatedly, I decided that I would use the unfolding of the song to try to articulate what I saw as the gift and challenge of Kathy's life and death.

I offer four lessons of how Kathy lived beauty awake.

The Art of Beholding the Sacred

To me, the first verse of the song is about the art of beholding the sacred or, to put it another way, the art of attention. Listen:

> *Let beauty awake in the morn from beautiful dreams,*
> *Beauty awake from rest!*
> *Let Beauty awake*
> *For Beauty's sake*
> *In the hour when the birds awake in the brake*
> *And the stars are yet bright in the west!*
> *Let beauty awake from rest*

The poet starts with everyday experiences that all of us share—morning, sunrise, dreams, rest. And he dares us to clothe everyday activities in beauty awake. Anyone who has sat quietly watching the sun's first kiss of the earth in the early morning knows the beauty of which the song speaks. And yet the song invites us to move beyond the spectacular one-off, awe-filled moment. Because beyond the spectacular lies the beauty of the mundane; that is beauty in everyday life. It is seeing and responding to beauty in every moment of the day, or at least as often as we can. I see this as the art of beholding the sacred.

Kathy was a genius at beholding others! She saw deep into you, her eyes touching your sacred beauty and good-ness. Kathy had a bold, quiet attentiveness. Anyone who got close to Kathy—no matter their age or social status, could feel the warm attentiveness of her gaze. Kathy knew her attention was like a watering can—whatever she gave her attention to would grow. She gave her atten-tion to others.

I think Kathy lived a beauty awake life because she recognized and beheld the beauty of others. Elizabeth Barrett Browning said, "Earth's crammed with heaven / And every common bush afire with God; / But only he who sees, takes off his shoes" (from Aurora Leigh).

This was Kathy—she was a shoe-taking-off kind of woman. She was one who truly saw deeply, beholding the sacredness of the everyday. Kathy knew and prac-ticed the art of beholding.

The Art of Dynamic Loving

In the second verse of the song, it is as if the poet starts again with the beauty of the common and the art of beholding, but then suggests that the art of beholding is not enough. If you want to follow the enfolding path of beauty awake, you need to go deeper. Seeing the sacred is not enough, you need to add the dynamic to and fro of the art of love. Listen:

Let Beauty awake in the eve from the slumber of day,
Awake in the crimson eve!
In the day's dusk end
When the shades ascend,
Let her wake to the kiss of a tender friend
To render again and receive!
Let beauty awake in the eve

Anyone who has been married for at least a year, knows that the dynamic giving and receiving of love is a messy business—where we are sometimes meeting each other and sometimes missing each other. This kind of dynamic love, which the poet calls rending and receiving, is always changing. If we want to live beauty awake, we have to learn the art of loving in the midst of ongoing change. This is no easy task. The art of dynamic love is about constantly learning to love anew.

Kathy knew about the art of dynamic love. She and Lyle were married far longer than a year—their journey together was a beautiful, messy journey of soulmates unleashed. Kathy knew more than her share of suffering and health issues. Consequently, she knew more than her share of prayer.

60

If Kathy were a song-writer, I think she could have written these words Leonard Cohen wrote at a time of grave illness:

If it be your will
That a voice be true
From this broken hill
I will sing to you
From this broken hill
All your praises they shall ring
If it be your will to let me sing.

Kathy did sing beautifully from her broken hill. As the world kept changing, she kept finding new ways to love those of us who had the huge gift of living alongside this dear woman.

The Art of Gardening Creation Blessed

To me, each new section of the song starts with a kind of implied critique. It is as if the poet is saying, *you like the art of beholding and the art of dynamic loving, well it is not enough.* If you want to live beauty awake, you have to go deeper. It is not enough to see deeply and love deeply.

The poet warns we cannot be bystanders of the sacred, only watching it and loving it. Rather the poet calls us to engage the world in the here and now. To touch the earth as creation blessed. To touch the earth and the world as sacred and holy, and then to transform this sacred soil into the beauty of the flower. Listen:

While we, the gardeners of creation blessed
Furrow the soil at our saviour's behest
And bury the seeds of our own life's death
And suffer God's glory to grow

Kathy was not a bystander of the sacred. Kathy was a gardener of the sacred. Where others sought the spotlight, Kathy loved as any had need. From the youngest to the oldest, Kathy loved all.

I've come to see the Parable of the Sower from scriptures (Matt 13:3-9) as a story about a wasteful gardener who keeps throwing seed where there is a very slim chance of success. What kind of gardener throws seed on the path, or rocky ground, or among the thorns?

Kathy was like this so-called wasteful gardener—planting seeds in love was more important than succeeding. Part of the way Kathy lived beauty awake was to seek out those who were suffering and simply be a loving presence in their midst. There were other ways Kathy was a gardener of the sacred: She helped plant and cultivate a bakery rooted in love and justice. (Tall Grass Prairie Bread Company is a local, organic bakery that pays its farmers and staff higher than average rates. Kathy helped start and sustain this bakery. Incidentally, my twin girls both work there). While Kathy was not a proud person, I think one of her favourite acts of gardening creation was helping to raise sons into men of love. Now, these are very advanced sacred gardening techniques—but Kathy was in love with her family. Ben and Dan, you are the living embodiment of your mother's art of sacred gardening.

Let Beauty Awake from Death

In this last verse, it seems to me that the poet tries to trick us. Having sucked us in with the beauty of sunrise and sunset, having taught us the art of beholding, the art of dynamic loving, the art of gardening creation blessed, the poet unveils the centre, the gift hidden in this journey. It's as if we have climbed the mountain and now get to see from the summit the secret of life. The big reveal: Let Beauty Awake from Death. Listen:

Let Beauty awake, in the morn from the cool of the grave,
Beauty awake from death;
Let Beauty awake,
For Jesus' sake,
In the hour when the angels their silence break
And the garden is bright with His Breath.
Let beauty awake from death

Lyle, Ben, and Dan, this is the chapter of Kathy that we are all still writing. Kathy lived her life as a profound example of Beauty Awake. But now, what of her death?

Listening to the song over and over, I started to fight with the poet.

Is death not the interruption of beauty awake? Isn't death the robber of beauty awake? Did we not pray that God would save Kathy and us from this day? Now, here in the presence of Kathy's dead body, among mourning friends and family, here you want me to say let beauty awake from death? Really? At first I was jealous of the song-writer. He ends his song, "Let beauty awake from death," but offers few clues as to what that means. How are we to hear those words today? The song offers nothing. "Let beauty awake from death," La, la, la, hum, hum. Sudden end. Thanks, Steve.

As I kept listening to the song, it was as if the poet whispered in my ear.

Did you not know this journey leads to death?

Did you not know that to live beauty awake you must also embrace beauty in death?

Then it was as if the poet whispered into my ear, almost mocking: *If you did not know this journey includes beauty from death, then go back to the beginning and see again with eyes of beauty awakening from death.*

Did I not point you to the sunrise and sunset?

Did I not give you this mini birth and death of sun everyday on the large screen of sky?

And did I not make both the birth and death of the sun

beautiful? Did I not give you the beautiful birthing and beautiful dying of the sun so that every day you could practice embracing the beauty of life and the beauty of death?

Did I not make you gardeners of this sacred soil so that every time you put your hands on this messy, dark soil, you could practice touching death and know that it is OK?

Did I not tell you to touch the soil of creation blessed, so that you would learn what every gardener knows to be true: there is no beauty of life without also the death of life—together created very good?

And so the chapter we are still writing about Kathy is about beauty from death. The challenge I think we are left with is, how can Kathy's way of living beauty awake provide us with guidance in embracing her dying in beauty awake? How do we take all the insights of her life and apply them to her death?

Tomorrow, as her body is laid back into the ground, she gets to return to this soil we call creation blessed. Often, as the body is laid to rest, someone speaks the words from Genesis: Ashes to ashes, dust to dust. Remember, these words are not a curse. They are a blessing and a dare to the living. You were created from the earth and to the earth you are intended to return. You were created from dust and to dust you shall return. Ashes to ashes, dust to dust. These words beg us to live our lives embracing our dustness, not as a curse but as a blessing of beauty awake. So that from the cool of the grave of our dear friend and sister, we can say with deep loving kindness: Let beauty awake from death.

Song Credits

"Let Beauty Awake"

Music by Steve Bell

Lyrics for stanzas one and two: Robert Louis Stevenson

Stanzas three and four: Steve Bell

Stanza five: Tom Wright

Chapter 8 - Embracing Dustness

 It's a kind of deep anxiety rooted in the fear
of disappointing others.

I was speaking to Rhona while taking our puppy, Kobi, on a walk through our neighbourhood. I was trying to communicate why walking the dog in our neighborhood had become stressful and anxiety-producing for me. Stress is not new to me but this kind of anxiety is new. When I walk the dog, I try to plot a path through our neighbourhood so that I will not run into anyone I know. This is quite difficult—and almost funny —as I have lived in the neighbourhood since I was eight years old! As I reflected on this anxiety, I realized it was not rooted in a fear of having to talk about Huntington's disease. I do that quite openly. Rather, it is a fear of letting others down. Growing up, I was a people-pleaser and overachiever. As Huntington's disease progresses, I am less able to please or achieve. My internal voice says, "Watch out. You will only disappoint them." I know I have great friends, and so this is not about them. It is entirely about the perceptions in my head.

As I was complaining to Rhona about how I let this social anxiety create a maze of barricades, we were interrupted. A man on the other side of the street was yelling and waving. I had never seen this man. But Rhona and I became completely silent. We both knew. From across the street, in a manner of seconds, we had both diagnosed this man with advanced stages of Huntington's. He was doing the Huntington's dance. (If you want to get a sense of what this looks like, check out this two-minute video and song, which I found online. It is called the Huntington's Dance:

https://www.youtube.com/watch?v=e50WiWgIbxg.)

The man we saw was largely non-verbal, could barely stand up, and was waving at us. His dog sat still beside him. As people passed by him on the other side of the street, we noticed he was welcoming everyone he met as a friend! We went and talked to him and confirmed our diagnosis and learned his name was Rob. We told him I also have the disease. There was a deep kindness in him.

Later that night, Rhona asked me, "So what did you think of seeing Rob today?"

"I was complaining of social anxiety and he was welcoming everyone he met. Ironic," I replied. I thought to myself that this man needs to be my teacher. He knew about compassion, freedom, embracing strangers, over-coming anxiety, and loving the world.

I reflected on the kind of wisdom that was present in Rob's way of being and I wondered how I could get past my anxiety to share in that wisdom. I was reminded of an exercise I had done with my university students in a class on non-violence, that I thought might help me in this task. In the non-violence class, we explored Gandhi's way of being and his statement that "the seeker after truth should be humbler than dust." To help my students become friends with that kind of imagination, I made them all write poems to try to unlock the wisdom of this statement. Realizing that writing poems requires a kind of willingness to be vulnerable, I decided that I should write my own poem. It reflects the spirit in which I wish to walk the path ahead, the way in which I hope to learn to be like Rob.

Embracing Dustness
Dust to dust
Ashes to ashes
This is no curse
Or last words of lament
It is a riddle key
To the way of Truth
It's a riddle key
To a life of nonviolence
The lover of truth

Embraces the way of the dust
The dust is free
Free from all striving
-to be on top
-to maintain control
-to become bigger and better
The dust does not consent
To the rules of the powerful
This non-consenting dustness
Transforms, even enemies
From below
it looks down on none
and can be crushed by any
And the one who can be crushed by any
Has defeated defeat
Winning and losing collapse
The dust-filled lover is hindered by neither
Humbler than dust
is the way of Truth
The lovers of truth embrace
the way of the dust

To many, embracing dust does not sound like true happiness. I think that to understand the true happiness that comes from this practice, you must give it a try. My experience is that embracing dust can teach us a lot about dancing with elephants and about true happiness.

There is a Swahili proverb, "When two elephants fight, it is the grass that suffers." The proverb communicates a

kind powerlessness that the grass feels when both domi-
nated and ignored by larger powers. But think of the
dust. The dust does not suffer in the same way as the
grass. The dust is an image of resilience that transcends
power and powerlessness.

If we are going to dance with elephants, we will get dirty.
If we see the dirt as a curse, we will never be happy. If
we see dirt as the way of dustness, then we can dance
with elephants and get dirty; we can still be people who
are truly happy.

Chapter 9 - Walking the Urban Pilgrimage

❦

Walking is a long-used mindfulness practice for those interested in a more healing and peaceful way. Mahatma Gandhi, Martin Luther King Jr, and Thich Nhat Hanh are well known for using walking in the service of building peace. However, they walked very differently from one another. It is a good thing they did not walk together! Gandhi would have won any race—he walked with speed, determination, and an inward, almost introverted focus. Martin Luther King Jr. would be second in a race. King walked as an extrovert, engaging others with a slow, pounding pace like a drum. Thich Nhat Hanh would be last in any walking race. With the speed of a tortoise, he would slowly take each step, as if it was his first and his last step to ever touch holy land.

Many spiritual traditions have some form of walking

pilgrimage as a way to awaken the heart and soul and to honor the sacred. For many in my circle of friends and acquaintances, *The Camino de Santiago* in Spain is the ultimate holy walking experience.

When I first went on long-term disability, I started walking. I had these voices of Gandhi and King and an image of sacred pilgrimage in mind. I also had in mind the voice of a Buddhist nun whom I had met during a visit to Plum Village—Thich Nhat Hanh's community. I asked what she thought was the most important mindfulness practice for non-Buddhists. To my surprise, she responded immediately: "Walking Meditation." So with these various voices in mind, I walked. Sometimes, these voices would fight with one another about the more sacred way to walk. But they found common cause when questions of *where* to walk arose.

Why do we need to go to the other side of the world to find sacred spaces? Such travel is the luxury of the rich and often the able-bodied. If we cannot touch and respond to the sacred in each step at home, what makes us think we will do better in some other place? If we do better in some other place, will it really help us walk each step, mindful of the sacred, when we return?

These questions led me to dare myself: Walk a sacred pilgrimage at home. Gandhi's famous Salt March was 386 km (240 miles) in 23 days—about 17 km a day. From having taught about Gandhi in my previous life as professor in peace and conflict studies, I also knew that when he returned to India, he went on a year-long journey to see every corner of India and learn how her people lived. So I combined these ideas. What if I walked every street in Winnipeg, to see how my neighbours lived? What if I walked this as an urban pilgrimage? Could I walk like Gandhi, or King, or Thich Nhat Hanh? Could I learn to walk as if each place were a sacred pilgrimage?

I bought a city map, a highlighter, and some refillable water bottles. I set out on my urban pilgrimage. I decided on a few guidelines for myself:

- No electronics—I did not want to be distracted. Phone, iPod, and all such devices would be left at home or in the car.
- No wallet—for a number of years I have felt awkward about mixing money and sacred practices. I had witnessed a number of Indigenous people doing Smudges. They would always take off their glasses, watches, and jewelry before washing themselves in the sacred smoke. I used a similar practice to symbolically take off my shoes to acknowledge that I was on holy ground. I did not literally take off my shoes, because while the ground was holy, it was also cold, since autumn was in full force.
- I would not talk publicly about my journey until I was more than 100 km into it. I loved the idea of the urban pilgrimage but I knew that I wanted

to speak from the perspective of practice rather than the realm of ideas. I told my family and a couple friends but no one else.

Beyond these few guidelines, I had no great directions. I just wanted to be present, to walk mindfully, and to enjoy touching the earth.

This was a beautiful time for me. I saw parts of Winnipeg I had never seen. Some days, I would contemplate a quote about walking. For example, I had heard the question: What is the speed of love? Response: Three miles/hr.–walking speed. But mostly, I tried not to fill my mind with too many thoughts and just go and be. This was energizing. At first it was hard for me to let go of my inner world of thoughts and emotions. But as I learned to broaden my horizon of interest, I had the time and space to cultivate relationships with people and places I would otherwise never have seen or met.

I highly recommend you set up your own approach to doing a pilgrimage where you are. If you want more teaching on walking meditation, I recommend Thich Nhat Hahn's, *How to Walk*. Learning to dance with elephants is in part about being on the move in a non-violent, non-harming way. Urban pilgrimage is a mindfulness training that touches on this kind of movement. I hope it will lead to true happiness for you.

Just as I reached the 100 km mark, three things happened that led me to give up my goal of walking every street in

Winnipeg. First, I got a parking ticket. This wasn't really relevant, but somehow it discouraged me. Second, Canadian winter arrived. Where we live, the winter temperatures go down to -40 C (also -40 F). Third, we got a puppy, which demanded a different kind of mindfulness training (the subject of the next chapter).

At some points, I felt like a failure. I had set a goal of walking every street in Winnipeg and I did not meet that goal. I had not walked as far as Gandhi's Salt March, which he did when he was over 60. I was 43. My competitive and goal-driven nature was still living strong inside me, and my inner voices told me I was a failure. Looking back, I see it differently, but it was not easy at the time.

Now my focus is less on covering every part of a map and more on simply taking each step in gratitude for life. This is a happiness project. The urban pilgrimage was the training ground that continues to shape who and how I am now.

Find some practice of walking meditation. It will probably look very different from mine. What matters is not how it looks, but rather the spirit you bring to it and your openness to learning to see anew.

Chapter 10 - Loving a Puppy

Tabitha prescribed a puppy for my family. Tabitha is an ex-Hutterite and co-owner of Tallgrass Prairie Bakery in Winnipeg. This is the same bakery Kathy Barkman (Chapter 7—Living Beauty Awake) helped start. Tabitha is also a friend and a member of our circle of caregiving friends (see Chapter 12—Responding to a Disease with a Circle). In our community, Tabitha is a bit of an Elder, meaning when she speaks, people pause to listen. At one of the meetings of our support circle (see Chapter 13), Tabitha took it upon herself to prescribe that we get a dog.

Later that night when we told our twin daughters what Tabitha had said, they were very excited. They had an ally. They had wanted a dog for years, and from time to time had tried to convince us. In fact, Sara had been working on a PowerPoint presentation to make her argument! Rhona knew that much of the work would fall on me, so she said it was my call. I am not entirely sure why I agreed. I had no sense that I needed to have a dog, but I respected the people who said it would be good for us.

We ended up getting a beautiful golden lab puppy. Koila picked him from the litter and Sara named him Kobi. And so our family expanded, in ways that none of us could have imagined. Kobi was born in December, 2014. Seven weeks later, we brought him home.

The first year we had some challenges as we slowly trained one another, but by now we are all in love with Kobi. Every day I hear my girls squeal in delight at how cute he is or how much they love him or how they will never find someone more handsome than Kobi.

To be honest, it is not just the girls who squeal in delight. Rhona and I get in our daily share of squeals—much to the chagrin of some of our friends and family.

Wake up—pet the dog, who calmly rolls on his back or leans in for a cuddle.

Go downstairs to let the dog outside and gently give—and take—some love on the way.

Before the coffee is made each morning, we have all participated in multiple acts of love and happiness.

Love is weird that way. It is not like money, which decreases as you use it. Nor is it like anger, which pushes others away as you use it. Love grows into more love.

Having a dog—even a poorly trained puppy—is minute to minute mindfulness training in happiness.

We've noticed this happiness is not contained to our family. Not everyone gets infected with this happiness virus, but as we walk down the street we see faces light up—children's, adults', people of all ages and abilities. I am not sure what people see when they see Kobi, but when he is present, smiles arise all around. It is profound. Kobi is a happiness virus.

Sometimes when people are having a hard time, they will pop into our house for some puppy therapy. Sometimes when the girls experience conflict or anxiety or are mad at their parents, they want to have Kobi around them. He makes us into better people.

There is a quote: "I hope I can be half the person my dog thinks I am." What I like about this saying is that dogs see us through the eyes of love. As long as we don't hurt them and attend to a few basic needs, the dog does not hold a grudge. Each time you walk through the door, he is just happy that you have arrived. And his happiness makes happiness arise within us.

Before Kobi, our family did not have any pets. I know many of you knew about the miracle of pets long before us. If mindfulness trainings are there to train us to love, then having a dog is one of the best mindfulness train-ings I have ever experienced.

For our girls, loving an animal so deeply has led them to

become vegan. When they saw our meat system as cruelty to animals like Kobi, they radically changed their diets. They recently had their one-year vegan anniversary.

Having a dog has helped us to let go of some fears and replace them with true happiness. A dog—and especially a puppy—is a lot of work. But as we let go of our need to have an always clean house, we have also increased our overall happiness.

To be an elephant dancer, you need to learn to love the elephant. If the elephant is too frightening, start with a dog. If you allow it, your dog will train you to increase your love and happiness.

Chapter 11 - Diving into an Ocean of Gratitude with Patch Adams

❦

Patch Adams estimates that, as a clown, he has been at 10,000 deathbeds. I asked him what he learned from being present at these deathbeds, dressed as a clown with toys in his pocket.

"They are not deathbeds," he said. "They are living beds. There are two states: alive and dead. From the second you are conceived, you are dying. That is not interesting —especially since you are also living."

Then he looked into my eyes and said, "Either you're living or you're dead. The fact that you are 'dying'— well, I see you as living. So where is the fun?" It was as if he was saying, you are living so live well and have some fun!

Later in our conversation, I asked him if, given his experience, he could offer a few hints on living well for those of us who are labeled with a disease.

"How many do you want?" he asked. Then he sat back and said, "We all die. Relax. The question is not 'how.' The question is: Are you living? Are you being the human being you want to be? Are your relationships healthy? Are you grateful? What is your sense of wonder? What's your sense of curiosity? What thrills you?

"You can decide to love life. You can decide to love your partner. You can decide to know what I mean when I say that a tree can stop your suffering."

Somehow, those words struck me as freeing. I don't need to figure out everything about dying. I need to keep living. To be thrilled, grateful, wonder-filled and curious about life and living. These are ways of being that are accessible to me.

If someone else had spoken these same words to me, they probably would not have had the same effect. Perhaps if I tell you some of Patch Adams' story, you too will feel a deep surge of gratitude for being alive and you might accept the deep dare to live a life shaped by caring for others.

Some people think they know Patch Adams' story because they saw Robin Williams portray him in the famous Hollywood movie. However, the real Patch

Adams is quick to point out that the film profoundly simplified and sanitized his life.

Patch was born in May 28, 1945. He grew up an army brat, following his father around the world and watching as war stole his father's soul. After his dad died, in 1961 during Patch's teen years, his mom moved the family to Virginia. This was a time of open racism. When Patch saw "Whites Only" signs on public drinking fountains, he came to believe that his country was fake and religion was fake because they allowed such injustice and dehumanization. As a teen, Patch was beaten up for standing against violence and racism. Over the course of a year, at the ages 17 and 18, he was hospitalized three times for attempted suicide. Patch did not want to live in world with so much violence and injustice.

It was during his third hospitalization that his life changed direction. For him, it was like a lightning strike: "You don't have to kill yourself. You need to make a revolution, a love revolution."

He was confronted by two questions:

1. *How do I find a love job for men in a capitalist system that is making its people sick?*
2. *How can I be an instrument of peace, justice and care every day?*

The first question set him on a quest to become a free

doctor. The second led him to practice clowning every day.

At the age of 18 he says he "dove into an ocean of gratitude and has never found the shore." At this same time, he identified six qualities that he committed to living everyday: happy, funny, loving, cooperative, creative, and thoughtful. He told me, "Since then, in 54 years, I never had a bad day!"

As a young adult, he turned his attention to books and to social experiments in loving, and playing. Through these social experiments, he crafted himself into an instrument of peace. He dressed in many costumes so that he could learn to engage people in theater. Every day for two years, he spent two hours calling wrong numbers to learn how to talk to strangers, trying to keep the other party on the phone. He also rode elevators, 10 hours a week in Washington, D.C., to learn the art of engagement.

For Patch, medical school seemed to teach everything that was wrong with society: elitism, racism, speed doctoring, medicine for money, hierarchy.

The year he graduated as a medical doctor, 1971, he also released an eight-page paper on a model hospital designed for holistic care. He called the model hospital Gesundheit! Institute.

For the next 12 years, a small group of families and doctors lived out a mini-version of the model to demonstrate that it could work.

Here are some of the striking characteristics of this model of care:

- No charge for medical appointments.
- Average patient visit lasts three to four hours, as opposed to the standard seven-and-a-half-minutes.
- All permanent staff live together communally.
- Everyone makes the same salary ($300 a month).
- Patients live alongside doctors and their families.
- No health insurance reimbursement.
- No malpractice insurance.
- Ecovillage environment. Eventually, the hospital bought 321 acres in West Virginia (the poorest state for health care), providing a place to soak in the beauty of nature with three waterfalls, caves, a four-acre lake, a mountain of hardwood trees, and wildlife.
- Organic farming on the premises; Patch was a goat herder for eight years.
- Integration of the healing arts.

When Patch started the mini Gesundheit! Institute, he and his colleagues thought the full-scale hospital would be built in four years, by 1975. Yet over the next 12 years, they did not get one donation. They learned that giving and loving were a kind of high. But they also learned that they would need to change their approach if they wanted to attract funds.

Patch then started to work full-time at outreach and speaking engagements to raise the money for the model hospital, a dream that is yet to be realized. You can donate here:

http://www.patchadams.org/donate/

He spends up to 300 days each year on the road and has visited more than 90 medical universities in 70 countries. Apart from doctoring, Patch finds he needs to have some ongoing way to care for others if he is to sustain his work. So he decided to responds to every letter written to him as an act of care. Further, he decided to make clowning trips into some of the neediest places in the world: war zones, refugee camps, orphanages, prisons, areas of abject poverty, and centers for veterans of war. In each place, he tries to infuse society with the joy of living. He sums up his approach by saying: "My spiritual path is loving people."

When I spoke to Patch over Skype, I saw a 71-year-old man dressed as a clown, with long white-and-blue hair that has not been cut since 1967. In characteristic style, his white mustache was curled up at the ends. He wore a pink-and-purple tie and bright red glasses to finish off the outfit. Across from me sat a man whose dream has not yet been accomplished, even after four decades of trying. But as he spoke, I knew this was an unimportant detail. He spoke with love, not bitterness.

Talking with Patch made me reflect on this question: What if the answer to most of our problems is to make others radiant? When we are not well, so many medical professionals tell us to focus on ourselves. But what if the key to our own happiness is to care for others?

From Patch, I want to learn the joy of living, the gift of living in gratitude, and the deep transformations that arise when we care and love those around us. This book outlines some of my own social experiments in loving, but Patch dared to me go further, bolder, and freer.

In my video recording of our conversation, you can hear Patch share his own story, as well as explore things like how a tree can stop your suffering, why loneliness is the worst human condition, and what tricks you can use to help people love and be joyful.

PART III
TRUE LOVE

Chapter 12 - Responding to a Disease with a Circle

You know the size of an earthquake by the violent impact of its tremors. When my mom was the same age as I am now, the year was 1990. I was in grade 12. We were probably about eight years into the earthquake of her Huntington's disease.

By then my parents' relationship had been crushed, piece by piece. My older brother—protecting himself by doing what I often wished I could do—got the hell out. My mom had already alienated herself from almost everyone. Much of the time, she stayed at home and would not answer the door. I was left alone, with her.

To make matters worse, I tried to be the compassionate, listening son, staying present through the trauma of the earthquake that knew no end. For my mom, those were the days of suicide threats and attempts. It was her I-hate-all-men phase and her eight-year-migraine headache phase and, to me, it was her you're-going-to-be-an-awful-parent phase. She spent most days in her house-coat, on the couch, throwing up into an empty four-litre ice cream pail, the kind she had previously filled with homemade chocolate chip cookies. Her cooking and baking days were behind her now. She was in the fog of Huntington's. We were all in the fog of Huntington's

She was still in denial that she had the disease. And we had 16 years of more earthquake trauma (and other things too) to go until she died.

Can I Stop Passing Down Trauma Earthquakes from One Generation to Another?

Mostly I try not to think about those days. But now I have this disease. Now my twin girls walk the same halls of our neighbourhood inner-city high school where I took refuge when I was their age. For some time now, each time my wife, Rhona and I argue, there is a moment when she looks at me in fear and sees a disease.

I keep wondering what kind of habits and supports could make this walk a little more bearable, maybe even enjoy-able, for my kids, Rhona, and me. I am reliving my teen years, wondering what might have helped us during the earthquake. Which ways of living, what kinds of mind-fulness training might equip us to live in a way that does not dump all the trauma of previous generations onto the heads of my girls? For me, loving those around me requires that I pursue that question with everything I can give.

I don't think we are ever alone, but as a teenager, I felt that way. In hindsight, I am still a bit jealous of my brother, who, while also caught in the earthquake, was always better at saying "no" and creating some distance. My mom, my brother and I needed support. Our circle was too small. Support was offered many times, but my mom was not interested.

So this time around, I want to try not to make all the same mistakes. I want to widen and strengthen our circle.

I have come to believe that people from various cultures have been gathering in circles for a long time. In Canada, gathering in circles to respond to traumatic events is quite common in Indigenous communities. Many of these practices were unjustly outlawed, shunned, and discouraged. But there is still a living memory among some of their elders. They remember ways that the community gathered in circles to try to help people walk in a healing way, to help people understand their identity and the connections to the world around them. I believe such practices were common around the world. Before states stole conflicts from communities, communities gathered together in circles to become strong again.

In my prior life as a peace researcher and teacher, I did a lot of work in the field of restorative justice. This is one of the settings where people around the world are re-learning how to use peacemaking circles to move from crime to community. Living Justice Press is a great book publisher whose single purpose is to share such examples of circle peacemaking.

Circles of Support and Accountability is an organization that powerfully developed circles around people who were incarcerated for sexual offences and who were held until the end of their sentence because of their high risk for reoffending. Keeping these offenders in prison until the end of their sentence actually makes our communities much less safe, as there's no transition and no accountability. People go straight from prison to the community, and because they have served their time, the state has lost the right to limit their freedoms or hold them accountable. Circles of Support and Account-ability steps into this problematic situation. The organi-zation has helped stop cycles of harm while helping some of the most problematic offenders find themselves again while surrounded by a community of care. The circle tries to offer support with reintegration into the community while at the same time creating account-ability by challenging behaviour that might lead to more harm.

This example has been a model for me as I have consid-ered how best to widen our circle and protect my family from the effects of the Huntington's earthquake. One of my greatest fears with Huntington's is that I will harm my own family, following the pattern of my mother.

Having spent my life exploring healing ways, I know that circles have great transforming possibilities.

As a family, we created a circle of support and accountability as a reference point for the journey. We picked six people from our church with whom we had a very positive relationship of respect. We chose people with the following traits:

- people with whom we could share freely;
- people from whom we would welcome support;
- people we allow to call out our bullshit; and
- people we welcome to help shape our family.

One of the things I like best about my church community is that through hard-won experience, the group tends to respond to traumatic events by creating circles of care. At life-stage changes, like turning 12, becoming married, and having children, the church gathers more naturally. But a similar approach is used for traumatic events: a breakdown of a marriage, the dying of a friend, deep conflict between members.

It is not a rule or requirement or even an expectation. It is simply done because people have witnessed firsthand the goodness that comes from sharing in each journey, especially at those most painful places of disorientation. So when a dear friend (and circle junkie) from our church offered to do whatever we wanted to make such a circle available for us, we agreed. We had already been talking and planning for such a circle.

We invited the carpenter, the artist, the baker, the psych nurse, the social worker, and the food justice advocate. I know, it sounds like a joke. But for us, these are simply our friends. Everyone said yes, even though each had many good reasons to say no. They are our companions. Right now, we gather every other month, alternating sharing circles and meals with kids. The carpenter facilitates.

Right now, we share our journey and build relationships of trust with every member of the family. We have also invited our circle to ask hard questions. Most nights turn into a conversation. Our friends have decided to educate themselves about Huntington's disease by going to conferences. One night we brought in the social worker for the Huntington's Society in our province. We discuss each member of the family and what support might be helpful. So many of my medical doctors are specialists in one part of my body. But the circle is different. This is holistic, offering support for the whole family. In time, they will hold me accountable to walk in a healing way. The work we do now has much to do with what they will be able to offer later.

The Wisdom of Circle Responses to Traumatic Journeys

I hope that sharing this journey with our circle of support and accountability takes some of the pressure off Rhona, my kids, and myself so that there is more space to enjoy the road ahead.

It seems to me that circles teach us a lot about living life with wisdom. So far, here are some of the gems I've learned:

We need one another. We often cannot heal or walk in a good way all on our own. We need communities of support and care to help remind us of our identity amid our disorientation.

Rather than trying to battle disease and trauma, circles provide a way to care for your disease, as if it were a crying child.

We respond to entrenched disagreement (the stuff we refuse to budge on) by eating meals together. Eating together is a sacred act.

You may be surprised by the kind of support that people are willing to give, if offered a concrete option like a circle. The gift of the circle extends outside its borders. Our twin girls both have jobs at the bakery that the Baker co-owns. Each month, we go on date night with a couple in the circle. Good things tend to happen as people are given permission to care.

When our circle first started to gather, our supporters were very aware that they did not know a lot about Huntington's disease.

In passing, we said that the national conference on Huntington's was coming to our city and that Rhona and I would go and see what we could learn. Without our knowing, members of the support group went to the church and asked for money for the whole circle, including us, to go to the conference to learn about Huntington's Disease. The church approved. Everyone from our circle signed up. When we all showed up for one of the main sessions, we filled a whole table! I should say we almost filled a table. One chair was left empty. Soon, someone we didn't know came and sat with us. We introduced ourselves. When our new friend learned that the whole table was from our church, and there for Rhona and I, she was shocked. She is a social worker who works for the Huntington Society of Canada. She commented several times on our odd arrangement. She said most individuals don't even get this much support from their family, never mind the wider community. That stuck with me.

Healing resources are out there. We often fail to find ways to access them. Creating a circle of support and accountability has benefited our lives. I am curious how others have created ways of accessing and engaging the communities around them to become circles of support and care. I encourage you to think of ways you might tap into the wisdom of the members of your circles.

When I got sick, a lot of people said, "If there is anything you need, let us know." I think they meant it. They didn't quite know what to offer and we didn't quite know what to ask. The circle gives us space to ask for specific help, but even when we say there is nothing we need right now, the response is always, "Don't wait until we gather again. Just call us."

For us, this kind of circle of intentional friends provides an ongoing way to face life with all its twists and turns. I hope you act on finding the wisdom resources of walking in a healing way.

Chapter 13 - Dying and Mourning with Love

⚜

We have been taught—by so many voices—to fear death. And yet death is so profoundly human. It is one of the few sacred tasks all humans share: birth and death. Often, but not always, it is these basic sacred tasks that unite humanity: breathing, eating, peeing, pooing, birthing and dying. Elephant dancers need to learn to perform each task with compassion and love. We need to resist the culture of fear and anxiety at each step. In fearing death, we often miss out on living and loving. Elephant dancers can use the dying of loved ones as mindfulness training on how to live and die well. Perhaps by learning to unlock the keys to dying, we will create the space to keep learning to love.

How do we unlock the keys to dying well? Here are some of my insights from mourning and celebrating the life of my mother-in-law, Kathleen Hildebrand, who died peacefully on September 22, 2016.

Does Every Death Need to Be a Tragedy?

While I was doing my master's degree in peace and conflict in Virginia, Rhona and I worked at a retirement community right next to the university campus. We were on call evenings and weekends to help residents deal with emergencies. Over time, we started to learn what was important to residents. They would often speak of dying. More specifically, they would speak of their hope to die quickly and relatively painlessly. For them, a quick death was living the dream, the best way to go.

When I reflect on the residents at the retirement home, I wonder about those who got their wish. I wonder if their families felt the freedom to celebrate this dream death. Generally, when someone dies we feel that we need to respond to the death as a tragedy. "I am so sorry for your loss," we say to mourners. And indeed, there is loss and sorrow that comes from death. But surely not every death is best labeled a tragedy. How do we create space to celebrate dying well, as a natural part of living? How do we let go of the idea that something was unfairly stolen from us?

Letting Go of Heaven

In Kathleen's last days, what did she fear? What made her anxious? In my view, one of things that made her anxious was her view of heaven, where she would be reunited with two husbands - the first had died of leukemia decades earlier and the second had died of cancer just three years ago. For her, the idea that she would die and go to heaven was not entirely a comforting thought—would she have to choose between husbands? This wasn't the dominant theme in her last days, but seemed to me to be consistently present.

As a Christian who has a degree in theology, I do not believe in a heaven that you go to when you die. I think that is a very dangerous idea that is not actually found in the Christian scriptures. This idea of heaven creates fear and anxiety for many people, and these are not the fruits of the spirit. The idea of heaven as a family reunion needs to be explored much more deeply—when was the idea invented? By whom? Who benefited from the idea? When it was put into practice, did the neighbours of Christians experience it as the fruits of the spirit: love, joy, peace, forbearance, kindness, goodness, faithfulness, gentleness, and self-control? If not, then the idea was likely not from God or from love.

It pained me to see Kathleen feeling confusion and anxiety about heaven when she needed her focus elsewhere.

The Power of Laughter, Tears, and Silence

Laughter, tears, and silence came like healing waves in the hospital room. They came again at home, at the viewings and at the funeral. This was a gift-the kind of gift that comes as family and community are present to the dying of a loved one. One of the many things I deeply love about my in-laws is that they are very comfortable engaging in all three sacred practices together: laughter, tears, and silence (not necessarily in that order). I think one of the keys to dying well is creating space and giving permission for these three healing friends to do their work.

The Wounded Healer

What did Kathleen care about? What was she curious about in her last days? I can't know with certainty, though I am bold enough to reflect on what seem to me to be the likely answers. After Kathleen died, I went to her condo. This was the week we were all supposed to help her move from condo life to assisted living. On the floor of her living room were empty boxes for moving. Of course, these would now be used to take away her last possessions. Her condo was not overflowing with clutter. Mostly, what remained were pictures of family.

I went and sat on her couch. On the coffee table were the TV remotes she could never figure out how to use without help. But the coffee table was mostly clean save for a book. I unthinkingly picked it up to see what she was reading. Knowing I was in a rural, conservative Bible-belt, I was not sure what I would find. I read the title, *Living with Huntington's Disease (A Book for Patients and Families)* by Dennis H. Phillips. She was reading about me! I flipped through the book—published by a university press in 1981. My mother-in-law, who was losing her vocabulary, was spending her last days trying to learn about my disease and what her family might be experiencing. In classic Alzheimer's style, she had kept reading and re-reading the same short section of the book and would then relay her "new" learning to other family members, again and again and again. But this moved me. Her attention did not focus for too long on herself. She was trying to help others. She wanted to understand me and my family.

This theme arose again later in the week when my wife and her siblings had to decide which charity they would ask people to donate money to in lieu of flowers. I was not at this meeting but was told afterward that the family wanted to pick something that reflected what Kathleen was interested in at the end of her life. They decided to ask people to donate to the Huntington Society of Canada. These were my in-laws who did not have Huntington's in their family, but as a last act of lovingkindness and sharing, they were asking people to donate to what might support my family. What a surprising act of kindness! It came in the midst of mourning, at a time when you wouldn't expect a family to reach out to support others!

Now when people say, "Sorry to hear about Rhona's mom-how are things?" I want to explain my deep sense of awe and gratitude, but in the moment words fail me. Perhaps I too am losing my vocabulary. I hope Kathleen's compassion and curiosity will guide me on this path.

Chapter 14 - Loving Our Ancestors

Our ancestors have much to teach us. In most cases, in addition to passing on wisdom, they may also have passed on trauma. Often, before we can benefit from them, we need to work on seeing our ancestors through the lens of compassionate understanding and, often, forgiveness. If we are going to work at loving our families, we need to look through the eyes of compassion at how they were trying—and some-times failing—to dance with the elephants in the room.

You can see for yourself one of the best examples of this kind of generational healing in a video called Hollow Water

https://www.youtube.com/watch?v=MMKIvv5p164

(4min and 49 seconds into this piece). The people in this community were some of the most inspiring people I've met in my travels and research around the world. Hollow Water is an Indigenous and Metis community in my home province of Manitoba. The people of Hollow Water were trying to interrupt the cycles of violence by focusing on sexual abuse—which had touched between 66 - 80% of the community. The video shows one of the first couples they worked with, and you'll see how they created a family tree of abuse as part of the healing process. Hollow Water is all about taking responsibility. They have learned to shift from blaming the individual; to instead, healing through the generations.

A great energy and focus arises when we learn that our task is to make sure the cycles of harm and abuse are not passed down to future generations.

I have experimented with applying this approach to my own healing journey. I worked back five generations. I think it would be great to go back seven, if I had that information. One of the insights of our Indigenous people is that to understand the violence now, we need to look back seven generations, and when deciding how to act now, we need to act in ways that benefit seven generations to come. I love this view.

I examined my family of origin, moving backward this way:

First generation: my children (and their future children)

Second generation: my siblings and cousins and I

Third generation: my parents and their siblings

Fourth generation: my grandparents on both sides of my family of origin

Fifth generation: my great grandparents

Then I considered the kinds of traumas they faced and the kinds of traumas they imposed on others. This will be different for every family, but here is my list.

SA = Sexually abused

PA = Physically abused

MA = Mentally abused

S = Suicide

SA = Suicide attempts

AO = Abused others

FG = First-generation immigrants (left a homeland)

IN = Institutionalized in asylums for the insane

ED = Eating disorder

D = Disease

A = Addiction (alcohol/drug abuse/gambling)

W1 = WWI

GD = Great Depression/Dirty Thirties (1929-39)

W2 = WWII (1939-45)

R1 = Voted for political parties that support genocide of

Indigenous people in Canada (Canada recently concluded a National Truth and Reconciliation Commission of the genocide treatment of its Indigenous peoples from 1876-1996.)

R2 = Would have a problem with their own child marrying someone from a different race

W = Treated women with less respect than men

WFB = Witnessed a family breakdown

WA = Witnessed community violence-atrocities

WT = Witnessed terrifying and perceived-to-be life-threatening event(s)

MH = Mental health issues

EP = Experienced poverty

DI = Divorced

Then I thought about each person in my family and tried to create a family tree of trauma. Of course, the tree is missing all sorts of very important information because there are lots of traumas that people do not speak openly about. But this tree does not need to be perfect in order to be healing.

Next, I tried to add as many of the indicators that I knew about and I asked relatives if they knew of other traumas experienced by our family. This process was very moving. Although I had intended to share my family tree with names removed, I've decided to keep it private;

even without names, it involves other people's stories that are not mine to share. But the point of this tree is to be inspired to break the cycles of violence and trauma instead of passing them down to the next generation.

Thich Nhat Hanh often addresses the topic of healing your ancestors. When I was at his community, each night they would practice Touching the Earth—a practice devoted in part to your ancestors. You can reflect on some of Thich Nhat Hanh's words by watching this video:

https://www.youtube.com/watch?v=2hg0CWwMvM8& t=145s. ("Touching the Earth" from Thich Nhat Hanh's book "Happiness

While I was in Plum Village, I modified this practice to fit my life. I had not yet made my family tree, but this is what I did: I went for a walk of healing for one ancestor at a time. It was important for me to touch the earth. In his book, *Happiness*, Thich Nhat Hanh says, "While touching the earth, breathe in all the strength and stability of the earth, and breathe out to release your clinging to any suffering." The earth is a healing helper. On each walk, I found a rock that I could hold in my hands to represent one of my ancestors. I walked slowly, thinking only about this ancestor.

- *What was your life like?*
- *What traumas did you experience?*
- *How did you see your other family members?*

- *What made you afraid?*
- *Who taught you fear and violence?*
- *Whom did you harm?*

Of course, we need to also ask about all the positives, but starting with their traumas helped awaken and open my heart toward them. So, with no real plan, I walked. Asking questions. Listening quietly. Sometimes I would go through the decades of that person's life. Sometimes I would breath in the strength and stability of the earth and then breathe out sufferings. When I found my mind racing with thoughts of unrelated things, I simply stopped walking. When I refocused, I took another step. This practice was not about distance or time, it was simply walking in a healing way with my ancestor. When I felt like I was finished, I would clutch the rock in my hand and make sure I was touching the earth: bare feet, sitting or lying face down. I said a prayer: "My dear ancestor, I know you suffered deeply. I bless you and wish you well. I let go of the suffering that is passed down through the generations so that our future genera-tions will thrive with compassion. My dear earth, please take these toxins and turn them into flowers." Then I would leave the rock in that spot. For me, this was very freeing. I do not mean to say that I am free of suffering passed on from past generations—I do have a genetic disease. But now I also have more compassion and greater happiness. Priceless.

The world is learning more and more about generational

trauma. These practices motivate me and equip me to not pass on as much of that trauma to future generations.

A related concept, but highly unexplored, is that of generational blessing. What are the blessings—the good things—that our ancestors passed on to us? What are the good things we will pass on to the next generations? But that is a topic for another time.

I have laid out for you how I am trying to work at five generations of healing. I don't have time to be frozen in bitterness by what the previous generations did or did not do. Healing is about letting go of the things that cannot give life and daily doing the things that can. The healing practices that work for you may well look quite different from the ones that work for me. But I do want to dare you to work at healing your ancestors.

Chapter 15 - Playing with Children

During the opening ceremonies of the Canadian Truth and Reconciliation Commission, I went to the sharing circle focused on the abuse that had taken place in residential schools run by churches and the government. There was an old Indigenous grandmother there. She came into the circle clutching the arm of a younger white woman. When the grandmother got up to speak, still clutching the arm of the young woman, she said, "I am so grateful to be able to draw on the energy and power of the younger generations. I do not know this woman but I must draw on her power to say what I must say today."

For me, children are just like this. Simply being close to them, perhaps even touching them, gives me energy, happiness, joy, love, and a will to live. Playing with children is a mindfulness training that leads to love. I have always liked kids, but now their presence is even more meaningful. In a social situation, if I can choose between playing with kids or talking to adults I don't know well, I will always choose the kids. Yes, for me this is the easier path, but it is more than that. Playing with children creates new, refreshing energy. When we are close to a baby, we can feel their gaze before we even touch them. Feeling their presence, we soften our own gaze. When they smile, we smile deep inside. Like some crazy quantum entanglement, we feel what they feel even if we are at a distance.

I adore my two teenage daughters. I probably get into more arguments with them than anyone else in the world. Of course, we each think the other is the source of the disagreements. And now there are more times when I get angry, which is a subject for another chapter. I mention this here just to say that we have all the ups and downs of the parent-child relationship, plus we must figure out how to relate to this elephant in the room called Huntington's disease. So life is complicated. Sometimes we completely miss each other. But I still adore them. I delight in them. I can't believe they came from me. When I hear one of them laughing out loud at some show on the internet—maybe even a show I would not choose for them—their laughter, most of the time, brings me deep joy.

Giving birth to children who might inherit a traumatic illness is controversial and needs to be thought through. In fact, with Huntington's disease, not having kids is encouraged by some. When we were in the United States and Rhona was pregnant, we were asked if we wanted to test the twin fetuses for the marker for Huntington's Disease, in which case we could abort the kids. We said no. There are now other options, such as implanting only fertilized eggs that do not have the Huntington's Disease gene. I understand the reasoning. If you could stop this trauma from being passed down through the generations, why wouldn't you? But for me to accept that logic, I would have to conclude that it would be better if I hadn't been born, which would mean that our daughters would not be alive, either (we don't know whether they have the gene or not). But I have loved living. If my life ended today, that would have been enough. And knowing that there are hard years ahead, it is still good. I love that my kids have also been able to live life. Even if their lives were cut short, radically short, I would not regret the life they lived. This is not to pass judgment on choices that work for other people. I am just saying that I am in love with my kids and I am deeply grateful for the life we have had and continue to have together. I draw energy from my kids. When I see how my daughters and nieces and nephews are living, I am emboldened to live well.

Chapter 16 - Being Disarming Joy
with Lucy Kalanithi

From Lucy and Paul Kalanithi, I need to learn how to be disarmed by joy. Paul died in March 2015 at the age of 37. A neurosurgeon and neuroscientist turned cancer patient, he spent his last year writing *When Breath Becomes Air*, which Lucy completed for him. The book has sold over a million copies since its release in January 2016.

After interviewing Lucy, I went for a long walk on the frozen lake near my cabin. I call it walking on water. It is here that I am sometimes able to hear the whispers of wisdom. Soaking in her story, it suddenly struck me: This is a story about being disarmed by joy.

Lucy Kalanithi is a medical doctor, Yale graduate, author, mother, twin, caregiver, widow, and Stanford faculty member. After her husband died of stage 4 lung cancer, she ensured his manuscript was published and wrote an epilogue. *When Breath Becomes Air* has been on *The New York Times* Best Sellers List continuously since its release. Did I say she is in her thirties?

When Breath Becomes Air offers lessons on living and dying with love and integrity, and should be on the core reading list of anyone who wishes to dance with elephants.

When I talked to Lucy, I asked why she thought the book had sold over a million copies. What resonates with people? What surprises them?

"The book is not only about dying. It is about living," she said. "Paul talked about this idea that life is not about avoiding suffering. People have been intrigued by our decision to have a child while he was terminally ill. When we were making that decision, I said to Paul, 'Don't you think having to say goodbye to a child will make dying even more painful for you?' Paul said, 'Wouldn't it be great if it did?' He was getting at that idea that holding joy and pain at the same time is a task for a lot of people. It is a task for all of us, really, at one point or another in our lives."

I know this to be true. Each time I share my story, I hear back from strangers who tell me that learning about my experience with terminal illness helps them to face surprises in life. The source of their challenges is different from mine. They wrestle with loneliness, the disorientation of age, caring for a parent with dementia, or even living with their kids. And yet we feel a connection that transcends our situations. I think we are connected because we are finding a good way to hold the joy and the pain together.

Lucy and Paul each seemed to have learned that there is a freedom in not trying to avoid suffering at all costs. That freedom is the freedom to live fully—not giving up, not just passing time, not withdrawing from life. The freedom to fully live is the willingness to experience deep joy even if it might be mixed with suffering.

Deeper into our conversation, Lucy told me, "I do not think Paul died feeling like he was losing everything. Paul died feeling like he had everything." He communicated this kind of joy for life that does not demand more. Paul worked on his manuscript until a couple of days before his death. His final words in the book are addressed to his infant daughter, Elizabeth Acadia. Those words powerfully communicate this deep, radiant joy that does not hunger for more. Lucy recited them to me:

> When you come to one of the many moments in life when you must give an account of yourself, provide a ledger of what you have been, and done, and meant to the world, do not, I pray, discount that you filled a dying man's days with a sated joy, a joy unknown to me in all my prior years, a joy that does not hunger for more and more, but rests, satisfied. In this time, right now, that is an enormous thing.

Paul was disarmed by joy. He was willing to taste joy, even if it led to great suffering in dying. And, to his surprise, he found a well of joy that was so quenching that he was never thirsty again. His joy came from beholding another with whom he was well pleased. Elephant dancers need to practice daily this kind of beholding another for which inextinguishable joy is a side effect.

It seems to me that for Lucy, being disarmed by joy took quite a different path. Paul's disarming joy, Elizabeth Acadia, is now in her terrible twos. While Paul rests, enfolded in the ground, Lucy and her daughter face life after Paul.

Lucy told me a story that I think sheds light on her different but similar path of being disarmed by joy. The Day of the Dead is a Mexican indigenous celebration, which Lucy said she did not want to misappropriate, but that she found so striking and so helpful. This is her story:

 The year Paul died, we were at the cemetery where he is buried. It's really beautiful there, overlooking the Pacific Ocean. On the Day of the Dead, the cemetery is a very active place of mourning, celebration, and participation. They have these tents for face-painting for the children and sugar skulls, like *calavera* skulls that you can decorate. They have a Mariachi band and a taco truck.

It is very striking to see that stuff in a cemetery, with all the colours and the paper flowers. There is just this intense juxtaposition of literally eating a taco while visiting Paul's grave and having all these kids around. It felt true to my own experience of life after Paul's death. The grief and loss and the memory of Paul and the pain of losing him were mixed with my continued love for him and the fact of life itself in all its colours. It is all blended together. I love that holiday.

Paul's unarming joy was a joy rooted in the life of another. For Lucy, joy comes from being able to see and respond to life's strange mixture of colours. Life did not unfold according to Lucy's dreams and hopes. But she is not bitter or angry or feeling like life is unfair. In fact, she is quite delightful to engage. I think she, too, is disarmed by joy. Disarmed by the joy of being able to see life for what it really is, to mourn for that which needs mourning and to celebrate the rich colours of life, sometimes in the same breath. This is a heart whose door is open. When compassionate eyes see life's joy and pain, the one disarmed by joy can still smile.

Lucy reminds me of a favorite poem by Thich Nhat Hanh, "Please Call Me by My True Names." This is just the end of the poem:

My joy is like Spring, so warm

it makes flowers bloom all over the Earth.
My pain is like a river of tears,
so vast it fills the four oceans.
Please call me by my true names,
so I can hear all my cries and laughter at once,
so I can see that my joy and pain are one.
Please call me by my true names,
so I can wake up
and the door of my heart
could be left open,
the door of compassion.

This poem is my prayer for all elephant dancers.

In my video recording with Lucy, she explores non-judgmental loving, rule-breaking, end-of-life care, the battle metaphor, the complexity of marriage and terminal illness, and other mindfulness tools.

PART IV
LOVING SPEECH AND DEEP LISTENING

Chapter 17 - Refusing to Battle My Disease

Battling disease seems like a bad idea to me. The idea that waging a battle against my body will someday lead to health strikes me as crazy. Why would we wish war on someone who already has a disease?

When I was told I had a terminal disease, the responses of my friends were telling. I know they were in mourning and that they had a deep desire that I would not have to walk this path. So many of them would say things like:

"Fight it."

"Find a way to get rid of it."

"We can battle this together."

"We will use all the weapons at our disposal."

They spoke from the heart and I took their words as a

kind of lovingkindness. But now as I continue on this road which some call chronic and fatal illness, I look back at the words of my friends and see that they are filled with military metaphors. Even the health care professionals spoke in the language of violence:

"…a misfolded protein is invading your body."

"Hopefully, research will eliminate the disease."

"Perhaps by destroying rogue cells…"

How strange! Just when I needed help to walk in a healing way, the people around me are turning to the language of war and violence. Now, this is not just my strange friends (though they are strange). This language of violence is everywhere in our communities. But something in me knew that metaphors of war would not help my journey of healing.

Those learning to dance with elephants need practice in deep listening. Not all the voices around us orient us to live in a reconciling and healing way. Sometimes even the voices of friends and health professionals unintentionally prod us down a path that cannot lead to health.

This chapter focuses on the mindfulness training of deep listening—listening for what lies beneath the surface, listening to distinguish that which can lead to good living from that which can't.

I did a little digging online to see who is thinking about this odd and pervasive "battle" perspective on disease and dying. The best I found was an article in the *Atlantic* titled, *The Trouble with Medicine's Metaphors* by Dhruv Khullar, M.D., a resident physician from Harvard Medical School. After surveying research on the topic, he concludes that military metaphors might cause more harm than good. What an understatement! Here are eight reasons I refuse to battle my disease (or use the language of war to find the path of love):

1. Battling My Disease Is a Losing Battle

With Huntington's disease, there is zero possibility of "winning the battle." The same is true for anyone with a fatal illness. I don't mean to alarm you, but all of us are in the same boat, as life is a fatal condition. We all "lose the battle" at some point. We are all supposed to fight but we are all losers! How is this helpful? Even just war theory says that a war cannot be just if there is no possibility of success. This is a war we should not be fighting.

If the choice is between winning or losing the battle, I am losing the battle. But I reject the choice.

I don't want to spend my limited energy fighting or battling anything. I want to enjoy the path.

2. Battling Disease Doesn't Work, Even for Those Who Win

People who "win" the battle with disease often still consider themselves losers. As more and more people

"survive" cancer, some of the "survivors" are rejecting
that label. They feel that the term does not shed light on
the many ways they are still affected by cancer and its
treatment. My wife's cousin is one such person. In fact,
she is working on a handbook to support people who
have survived cancer but have not been able to return to
their previous level of functioning. More research is
coming out on this topic. Livestrong's research shows
that 98% [of cancer survivors] experience continued
physical, emotional, and practical concerns. Yet many
did not receive help for their needs. Even in actual wars,
we are finding that soldiers who've "won" the battle
have high rates of suicide, PTSD, depression, and
domestic violence. If that's what winning the battle looks
like, I don't want any part of it.

3. Disease Is a War Without an Enemy

Medical studies show that those who approach their
disease as an "enemy" tend to have higher levels of
depression and anxiety and poorer quality of life than
those who ascribe a more positive meaning. They also
tend to report higher pain scores and lower coping
scores. I used to teach peacebuilders how to diminish
their enemies by not cultivating them in the first place
and by loving them in the second place. It is remarkable
to me now to see medical scientists make the same claim
about health! Enemies are not good for us. If I must
battle my disease, I make an enemy of my body. No,
thank you.

4. Battling My Disease Feeds Denial

"Your mom took denial to a whole new level." These words came from my Huntington's disease health team. My mother had only one tool: denial. For those of us around her, this denial created a wake of misery. I vowed not to repeat that pattern. Over the years, I have developed a nose for sniffing out denial. I have learned that I need to be careful when people tell me that I should be free of this disease. I try to receive these comments as good wishes. But if I let myself, I can start thinking, *maybe there is a way to get rid of this. Maybe some prayer, some action, some science...will free me.* For me, the path of denial leaves an empty space where misery can grow, especially in those around me. If I pretend I don't have the disease or that I will get rid of it, then I pay less attention to living each moment with care. For me, the battle image feeds denial. I think this is very dangerous for my family.

5. Battling Disease Is Inspired by a Violent, Colonial, Macho, Paternalistic View of the World

Shortly after Justin Trudeau was elected as Prime Minister of Canada, he was asked why his cabinet has an equal number of men and women. He responded, to the cheers of crowds, "Because it is 2015." In the same way, I feel it is passed the time to be done with the violence, oppression, and discrimination embedded in our culture. There is something about the European-

Caucasian way of being that has allowed violence and oppression to touch every aspect of our lives: in medicine, politics, theology, and criminology. *Uhh, let's find the problem and kick the shit out of it. Uhh, let's kill the Indian in the child. Uhh, God demands bloody punishment. Uhh, what criminals need is more pain and suffering.*

Canada recently had a Truth and Reconciliation commission. We agreed to work to get rid of the very imagination that inspires the grotesque ways we relate to Indigenous peoples. The path of reconciliation must include exploring how violent oppression informs all areas, including medicine, politics, theology, and criminology. So, what does an approach to medicine look like post-Truth and Reconciliation? We must let go of find-problem-and-kill-it medicine. We must let go of violence-inspired medicine. Battling my disease is not for me. I put my hope in embracing dustness.

6. Battling My Disease Serves as a Blinder

Nobel Prizes have been awarded to scientists for rejecting a strictly mechanical understanding of life. The machine metaphor was a huge blinder for them. With the blinder removed, they could make revolutionary advances in fields such as neuroscience, quantum physics, and organizational leadership. Likewise, our assumptions about the need for violence blind us to the wisdom of old and the wisdom yet to come. We miss the wisdom of other traditions. I'm letting go of the blinders and looking for wisdom wherever I find it.

7. Battling My Disease Does Not Help Me Practice Loving Speech or Deep Listening

Those of us trying to practice loving speech and deep listening know that the way of violence does not lead to the way of healing, particularly in situations where the potential for violence already exists. Increased aggression is a very common symptom of Huntington's, especially for men in the first stage of the disease. The incidence of domestic violence is a lot higher than average in Huntington's families. So far I have not done this. But this increase in aggression is not unique to Huntington's. It is very common with many mental health issues and chronic conditions. If we are going to stop traumatizing our families with the fallout of violence and aggression, we need to stop promoting violence to tackle disease. Rather than telling me to battle a disease, ask me how things are going with practicing loving speech or deep listening. I need this mindfulness training to protect my family.

I hope I have made it clear that the battle metaphor seems completely unhelpful to me. Dancing with elephants seems to me to be a better metaphor, one that allows us to engage with that which we fear without adding more violence to the equation. We need to do everything we can to avoid the way of violence. Cultivating deep listening, loving speech, and a dark sense of humour can help. We also need the support of our friends, families, and health professionals to avoid the path of violence while at the same time cultivating a more healing path.

Chapter 18 - Naming Your Own Way

One evening several years ago, when I was putting one of my then nine-year-old twins to bed, she looked up at me and said, "Dad, why do they call it Huntington's disease?" I responded, "What do you think they should call it?" She said, "Huntington's disease sounds too scary. They should call it Starburst." At the time, I leaned over and said to her, "Well, if they called it Starburst, everyone would want to have it!" We had a good laugh. At a young age my daughter knew the power of claiming the space to name our own experience, despite what doctors might tell us. This was not the first time I had learned this lesson.

Naming, done well, is an overlooked and underused mindfulness training for elephant dancers. It is a form of loving speech that arises from deep listening.

They Call Me a Rape

Years ago, a rape victim taught me a similar lesson about the power of naming. Rob Baum's poem powerfully communicates how naming creates and defines experience. Here are just two lines:

They call me a rape
but I say it was done to me

The criminal justice system begins by naming the harm according to its own standards and not according to the experience of the victim. "They call me a rape." The victim is sidelined, or, as Rob Baum's poem goes on to explore, "neatly transcribed and tucked in sweet dreams amid the files...already I am textbook material."

Sometimes I feel like the sidelined victim given the external label, objectified, and struggling to find space to define my own experience. I don't want to be considered nothing more than my disease. I want to name my own experience, rather than taking the definitions of the medical field. I am not against the medical sciences. I know that, like many others, I stand to benefit from them. However, I don't want to be robbed of this important task of naming my own experience. If my daughter knows the deflating power of being called a disease, I should not think I can ignore this insight without causing more harm.

The First Sacred Tasks

In the Christian sacred texts of my own tradition, the first tasks of humanity were breathing, eating, and caring for creation. I think these sacred practices are often over-looked, especially in most Christian traditions. But it is the next sacred task that caught my imagination. According to this creation story, God sees that humans are bored. God seeks to create partners for humanity and creates all the wild animals and invites humanity to name them. This is not the kind of naming intended to control or dominate. It is much more sacred and intimate. It is the kind naming that allows the namer to be freed from boredom by recognizing the connection, distinction, and partnership of the other. It seems to me that this is more like the way I name my lover than like the way a Lord might name his subjects. Perhaps this kind of love-naming should be a core practice for living. What would a community, or even a person's life look like if it were formed by these sacred tasks: breathing, eating, caring for creation, and love-naming?

If I were to guess the lessons in the creation story for me, I would think that claiming the right to love-name my own path and experience might be important. "Being a disease" might cut me off from community. *He is not normal, not like us.* Being labeled with a disease might create a dis-ease of loving partnership. In the creation story of my tradition, isolation, boredom, being cut off from community, and lacking loving partnerships are all part of the problem because they do not orienting us toward a healthy way of living in the community.

What Do You Do for Work?

I have not yet found a good answer to this question. Usually I tell people I am on long-term disability; sometimes I tell them I used to be a university professor. Most people respond with regret, awkwardness, and sometimes sympathy. I don't blame them. It is like they fell into a trap. One of the key ways we get to know people is by asking about their job. But what about those of us who can't work? Sometimes I take some delight in how people squirm when I mention long-term disability. Some even take a step back, perhaps trying to protect themselves in case what I have is contagious. Other times I get caught in my own feelings—it is like the walls go up and I get cut off from friendship. Curiosity is replaced by pity. What am I going to do with all this pity?

Then I noticed that naming my career as long-term disability is like letting others name me a disease. These are frames of reference for my life which seem to be leading to pity, despair, and disconnection. What are my options for re-framing? How could I name my situation in a way that leads to healing?

Here is one option:

> New friend: Jarem, so what do you do for work?
>
> Jarem: Well, it is a bit embarrassing! A few years ago, I won the lottery.
>
> New friend: Wow. How much?
>
> Jarem: $1.14 million (that is the sum of my monthly disability payments over 25 years, which is the upper life expectancy for someone with Huntington's disease)!
>
> New friend: Do you want to party?

Pity is replaced with partying! What a transformation. Lottery winner or long-term disability? Hmmm....

I like how winning the lottery is rooted in part of the truth and re-frames disability toward living life. However, there is a lot that I don't like about the winning the lottery answer—it reduces life to money, it denies the difficult journey ahead, and it doesn't help the people around me to engage in the journey I am on.

I don't yet have a name for this journey. For me, right now, elephant dancing works. This task is deeply personal. It is my hope that each of us keeps naming and renaming the journey of stumbling toward a more healing way.

Chapter 19 - Making Friends with Darkness

66 Your uncle spends most of his time huddled in darkness, in a quiet room with a thick blanket covering his body.

I have been unable to get that picture of my uncle, in the advanced stages of the disease, out of my mind. How do I prepare myself for this future?

Once you decide to embrace darkness, a different world comes into focus. I find this world more mysterious and more beautiful. Most of life begins in darkness. A seed falls into the ground, and dies. This is where life begins again: in the darkness of the soil. Light is important. We could not exist without the sun. But darkness is also important. We cannot exist without it. Plants can't exist. Babies can't be born. People can't sleep. Life as we know it would end if we had no darkness. So if we look at the soil or at the womb of a pregnant mother, we see that we need the warm embrace of darkness for life to flourish.

Now when I think about my uncle, maybe he was returning to the womb. In a fetal position, encased in the womb of a blanket, he lies in the stillness of the dark. Huntington's disease returns you to infancy—limbs moving involuntarily, completely dependent. Some Indigenous people say that old people have this tendency to return to the fetal position—that is why they walk all hunched over.

Experiments in Embracing Darkness

I have taken on some experiments to help me reframe the memory of my uncle into something more positive. I have been working at readjusting my approach to darkness. If you would also like to experiment with darkness, here's how you can give it a try:

Sit in complete darkness and silence for 30 minutes at a time. If you must think about something, think about the womb and the ground you return to after death. Extend as you wish. Repeat as necessary.

Or lie in bed in the fetal position, under the covers, in complete darkness and silence for 30 minutes. If you must think about something, think about my uncle craving this still darkness. Repeat as necessary.

There are some things that can only be experienced in

silence and darkness. Now I anticipate sitting in darkness. It feels like it enfolds me. I can feel the hairs on my skin relax as they receive the darkness like a thick blanket. Overstimulation is everywhere. To me, it feels like strong wind on raw flesh. But darkness and silence have become good friends of mine. I can reside in darkness. I can build a home in darkness. I can abide in darkness. In this stillness, I find my home.

Perhaps I understand my uncle now. Beneath it all, there is a deep yearning for peace. But it is more than a yearning. A yearning marks the absence of something. Those who have made friends with darkness and stillness know my uncle discovered a way to experience the fullness of peace.

Chapter 20 - Remembering Forgetting Is OK

❦

One day I lost my wallet—three times! Each time, I retraced my steps to try to find it. I found it once in the Safeway parking lot. I must have looked like I was searching for a bomb as I ran around the parking lot looking under cars.

I found it another time in a great little local grocery store. One of the employees who was outside having a smoke saw me doing my car-to-car bomb run and asked what I was looking for. He was leaning against a fence just off the store's property. I told him. He pointed at the fence post. My gaze turned up from the parking lot to see that someone had neatly placed the wallet on the post. I am grateful for smokers.

The third time, my wallet had fallen out of my pocket while driving and slid under the driver's seat. That was all just in one day. No joke. No, nothing was taken from my wallet.

I am not only talented at losing wallets, I am also good at losing iPhones. I think I've lost my phone three times now, though not all in the same day. A couple of times, Rhona received texts from random strangers telling us where to pick up the phone. I'm learning this is a good way to meet the neighbours. One time, a woman said she found my phone right in the middle of the street by the local elementary school, just after school was let out. One time, I lost it with the battery dead. After a couple days, I used "find my iPhone." It was in a store I had been to earlier that week. The employees noticed the phone was dead so they charged it just in case someone tried to figure out where it was. Each time, it has been returned in perfect condition. Oh, yeah, there was another time I left it out overnight in the rain. That one died. Now our family rule is that I get the oldest hand-me-down phone we have.

I am not bragging. I am just trying to show that remembering is an hourly activity for me. Sometimes I succeed. Sometimes I don't. Before I was sick with Huntington's, losing my wallet would upset me and throw me for a loop. But with Huntington's, my view has changed. Now, instead of going into a rage, I get to meet the friendly neighbours!

At some stage, my forgetting could endanger my health or the health of those around me (e.g leaving an stove element turned on). At that point, I still think forgetting will be okay but I will also need to trust my community of caregivers when they say it is time to make different living arrangements. I've recorded this hope in this book, so in the event that I forget, please just show me this page!

If I am going to have to work through anger, frustration, and anxiety every time I forget something, I will have no time to do anything else. I do not want my days to be full of anger.

So if you see me touching myself oddly when leaving the house or walking down the street or coming out of the store— know that it is not what you think. *To try to not forget*, I tell myself. *Remember the trinity*. Then I touch myself, doing what might look like the sign of the cross: wallet, keys, and phone.

When I do forget, most of the time I am going to be kind with myself. I can smile and say there is more of that to come. When others forget things, I tell them we are part of the same club.

Now, for some, finding themselves forgetting is a painful thing. I know what it is like to wonder if your forgetfulness is an early symptom of something more serious. For Rhona's mom, part of having Alzheimer's meant that she forgot all the time. Forgetting was one of the few things she would remember to do. But that was fine. She would usually say, "I should remember." I always wanted to shout out, "Stop 'should-ing' yourself. Your brain is not working." Memory comes and goes. Ironically, the more angry or anxious you get, the worse your memory works.

So, whatever you are facing—be it aging or traumatic disease or some other elephant—please pledge not to fill your days with anger by getting mad at your memory. The people around you do not need your anger. They need your loving presence.

Chapter 21 - Breathing Anger

Anger is something I wrestle with. Ask my daughters or my wife. They know that sometimes I get mad and it takes quite some time to cool down. To make matters worse, anger has not traditionally been my thing. It is in the last decade and a half that I have had to wrestle with anger.

The problem is not anger itself, but rather the ghost of my mother. Her ghost haunts us. I don't mean I've seen some version of Casper the ghost. I mean that hollow silhouette that my mother became still haunts us. If you were to ask Rhona what she fears, what her elephant in the room looks like, she would tell you that she fears me becoming like my mom. Or at least the person she got to know when we were married, nine years before my mother died.

As Huntington's disease progressed within my mother,

she started to fixate on things that made her angry. For example, when our girls were born in 2001, my mom learned that we had given Sara the middle name of Rhona's mother. She decided it was not fair that our other daughter, Koila, did not have her name. This led to months of agony for all of us, as my mother would leave 25 messages in a day, on my work phone, demanding we legally change the name of our daughter.

Anger +Fixation = Agony

Sometimes, I get jealous of the people around me who don't come from Huntington's families. Many of them get angry but don't have to worry about being haunted by a mother with Huntington's. But when I am more clear-sighted, I see that anger is a toxin for all of us—those of us with Huntington's Disease and those without.

In the hopes of learning more about letting go of the toxins of anger, I share here the practices I have been experimenting with.

Time Outs for Breathing

It used to be our children who got the time outs. Now it is me. I give myself time outs. When I can feel the temperatures rising, I explain that I need some space and go up to my room. This does not always solve the issue but gives me space for perspective and breathing. Some-times I lie on my back on the floor and try to practice mindful breathing. Sometimes I can slow down and even enjoy taking breaths of life. Then the joy of life and breath tends to dissipate the anger. Others times, this does not work at all.

Mantras

Thich Nhat Hanh taught members of his community to use mantras to remind themselves to act with compassion when doing everyday things. For example, before starting a car, the monks and nuns are supposed to say, "When the car goes fast, I go fast." It is a kind of reminder to act responsibly with the car. Incidentally, at least one of the nuns—the one who picked us up from the train station—seemed to see this mantra as a dare to go crazy fast. Mantras probably work best when you make them for yourself. Mine have changed over time. At one point, when I was regularly getting upset, I set out to create a mantra. The only one I could come up with was, "I will not return evil with evil." It is a line in Christian scriptures which speaks to not returning violence with violence. To be honest, though, part of what I liked about it was that I could still imagine that whoever I was mad at was doing evil to me and I was going to act better than them. This mantra was a judgment of others and was certainly not ideal, but it did help me through a rough time. I would use it to remind myself that I was not going to add anger to anger. I never said it out loud.

Here are some other mantras I have used over time:

- *We have bigger fish to fry.*
- *How do you want the girls to remember you?*
- *How can we be guided by loving speech and deep listening?*

These can be helpful when they act like little bells reminding us to be loving to those around us.

A Cabin by a Lake

We've only had the cabin a little over a year. I know this is not financially possible for most. I share it because it has been fantastic for our family. We have a place where Rhona and I can go at the drop of a hat. In a year's time, when the girls are driving, they may also decide they too need an oasis of beauty where they can soak in sustained times of silence, reflection, and darkness. For me, the quiet and the darkness at the cabin feel like being soaked in healing balms.

Do Things that Create Joy and Love

We each need to regularly do things that create joy and love within us. If we want to offer joy and love to one another, we need to build up some excess love. Ask yourself and the people around you, what actions create joy and love within you? Pledge to make sure to do those things regularly. Everyone will be happier.

Listen for the Symphony of Creation

Go outside. Taste the air. Touch a river. Find some grass. Stand in the presence of the trees. It can do wonders for you.

Anger and Power

When I was first getting to know Ovide Mercredi, a Cree and a former National Chief of the Assembly of First Nations, we went for a long drive to talk, mostly so that he could poke and prod me, to see if we were a good fit. One of the things he taught me about on that first drive was anger. He said he was working with young Indigenous men to move beyond their anger. He explained that they had a right to their anger. Anger is a right response to injustice. But what he had to teach them was that every time they expressed their anger publicly, they lost their power and their voice. The public sees "just an angry Indian," he said. He was trying to teach them to see what lies underneath, deeper than anger. I know when I get angry, I too lose my power and my voice. Rhona and the girls most often think my anger is a Huntington's symptom. Every time I let my anger out, they don't hear my words or my concerns.

Reflecting on Ovide's insights about anger led me to write this poem:

The Freedom of Non-Entitlement

Beneath some of my suffering lies anger
Beneath anger, impatience
Beneath impatience, entitlement and wrong expectation

Entitlement is the seedbed of wrong expectation
Expecting now what cannot be now creates impatience
Impatience erases time and creates anger rooted in the
injustice that our wrong expectations cannot be
lived now
Anger overflows to suffering
The suffering of wrong thinking and
The suffering of wrong action
The presence of this kind of suffering
waters the seeds of anger, impatience, wrong expectation
and entitlement
And the cycle of violence goes on

Transform entitlement and a new horizon of being
Bubbles forth into the present moment

Through the law of non-entitlement
we can embrace and enjoy death
The ones who know
the universe does not owe them anything
are free
A great weight is lifted
We are not entitled to our entitlements
They are not what makes us beautiful

The flower follows the law of non-entitlement

It does not expect to live without end
It does not see its own death as injustice

Gazing at the flower we know will die
Does not feed within us the seeds of anger
Somehow suffering diminishes
in the presence of the flower's fragile beauty

How can I live and die
Like the presence of the flower?
How do I embrace the way of non-entitlement?

Chapter 22 - Practicing Awe During Winter's Creeping with John Paul Lederach

John Paul Lederach is one of the most accomplished scholar-practitioners in the field of conflict transformation and peacebuilding. He has spent his life trying to help others walk in a more healing way. Eight years ago his wife, Wendy, was diagnosed with Parkinson's disease.

In my search for a more healing and loving way to face disease, I needed to seek out someone who understood my approach to peace, conflict, and change while at the same time understanding the challenges and gifts of a long, slow, progressive disease. I knew I needed to seek out John Paul, who was one of my favorite professors when I was completing my master's degree at Eastern Mennonite University in Virginia. When Wendy was diagnosed with Parkinson's, I was dealing with learning that I would get Huntington's disease. There are a number of similarities between the diseases, including the slow decline toward death, which can be as long as 25 years. I wanted to see what they were learning about facing disease.

John Paul is the author of more than 20 books on conflict transformation and peacebuilding, including one published by University of Oxford Press. What I find more interesting about him is that his work took him to places like Nepal, the Philippines, Columbia, West Africa, East Africa, Nicaragua, Northern Ireland, and Spain. He often stayed involved in these places for decades. He is a modest, engaging, and profoundly curious person who does not shy away from the complexity of life. He even has a sense of humour. For example, he likes to point out that he used to specialize in church conflict but that was too hard, so he moved to settings of long-term violence.

Wendy, I've known only from a distance. She co-founded a Ten Thousand Villages retail store in Harrisonburg and ran her own jewelry line later with artisans in the developing world. As far as I could tell, she was a ball of positive energy and a good person.

I was delighted when John Paul agreed to let me interview him for my video series. After some warm words, he jumped right in. Here are a few snippets:

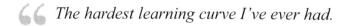 *The hardest learning curve I've ever had.*

It is like a new landscape you've never walked.

It comes into life unannounced.

It is not easy.

We're floating in a world that is less than visible.

I have failed amicably and I am still learning.

I've discovered that my well was not very deep.

This is not a disease that is a lightning strike like cancer. It is like winter creeping in.

It's like a slow violence, kind of like climate change. We all know it is there but because it is slow and the time frame is large, we don't notice and respond as we should.

I liked hearing these words. I do not take joy in the pain felt by another, but I take comfort in honest, open reflection. My teacher was not going to pretend to have all the answers. He did not hold himself up as a perfect caregiver for Wendy, even as wanting to be a good caregiver.

Winter had come for them. And as in the TV show *Game of Thrones*, winter is not about to go away anytime soon. All the peace and conflict transformation skills could not hold off winter. But one of the things John Paul and I share is the knowledge that peace is the way we struggle. Peace is not the absence of the storm. Peace is not some tranquil, idyllic place. And peace does not keep winter at bay. But peace names the way we struggle with that which lies before us.

We discussed what helped and what did not help from our academic field and from our shared Mennonite background. John Paul added to something we had observed: many of the practices of faith communities are held in communal settings. When it is hard to be around large groups, communal acts no longer serve those facing this kind of disease.

Then he offered me a gem. John Paul loves telling stories, so here he is in his own words:

> *Faith is also about a sense of awe that is captured in the mystery of the extraordinary gift of life and the world we were born into. Nature often brings that for me. So a lot of my faith practices have been less communal and more about an in-depth conversation or through the daily dose of vitamin awe. We need a daily dose of vitamin awe. We tend to see awe as something that we experience once a year. We go on vacation. But think about what you did this morning. You told me you "walked on water this morning"* [walking on a frozen river, at -40°C/F with my dog]. *That tells me you are a person who*

has been nurturing your daily dose of vitamin awe. I don't know why we don't have that as a core practice. To be very honest, if I experience awe in the congregational setting, it is almost always around singing. Singing together is something that captures awe, and it has always been there. When we're singing, we lose sight of all our differences, which really is an amazing phenomenon.

I think one of the big challenges is how not to become callous or cynical or bitter.

Callous means you do things that just keep the pain at bay—you're not going to be touched by this thing. Cynical means that you might use all sorts of defences to avoid going very deep into how painful this is. And bitterness comes when you know how painful it is and you are angry.

I don't think there are a lot of remedies for the winter creep other than vitamin awe. With vitamin awe, everything pops open and becomes alive again.

Cultivating awe is a form of mindfulness. Awe is there and present in almost everything around us every day, but we so rarely touch it.

I left the conversation feeling hopeful. This isn't a hope

that arises out of ignorance or wishful thinking. There is a much stronger hope that arises when we learn how those living in winter find ways to delight in the present moment. Going to church may no longer work for me. However, John Paul points toward the practice of seeing and responding to awe every day. Even I can do that.

Wendy's emails always come with a signature line: "When you stumble, just make it part of the dance." In some ways, she is teaching people the same practice of cultivating awe. We cannot stop the stumbling. But if we are not filled with fear, we can make the stumbling part of the dance. Awe is still available, amid the creeping of winter.

In my video recording with John Paul, he reflects on the gift and challenge of slowing down, becoming an artist of change, being surprised by impatience, sustaining curiosity, poetic listening, and the gift of quality presence, which he calls "alongsideness."

PART V
NOURISHMENT AND HEALING

Chapter 23 - Embracing Weakness

"We have heard nothing from you for six months. What has happened? Has your disease made it impossible for you to continue to write? How are you? Are you doing okay?" These are the questions I have received from my friends when they haven't heard from me in a while.

Don't cry for me, my friends. I have been enjoying practicing the embracing of weaknesses—more specifically, how to rock tunnel vision. While the "successful" strive for an endless stream of multitasking, I have been (re)exploring the one-thing-at-a-time method. Aging and my Huntington's disease have combined to strip me of any illusion that I might be able to multitask my way to anywhere.

In the "normal world," people expect multitasking. We are expected to get things done while at the same time responding to waves of emails, Facebook posts, phone calls, tweets, newsfeeds...

But I have been learning to lean into what I saw as my weakness and that which I feared. I have a one-track mind. And I am celebrating it. I have a deep, burning desire to focus all my attention on one thing until it is finished. Rather than fight this, I experiment with living into it. I have completed a number of big tasks this way: painting our cabin, creating a book and a blog, refinishing the kitchen, redoing hardwood floors. However, to do this, I have had to ignore everything else. I don't respond to friends and family. I don't pay bills. I don't clean the home. I avoid all social settings....

Elephant dancers need to embrace weakness if they are to flourish. Therefore, I am sharing with you four secrets to rocking tunnel vision - or whatever it is that you fear within yourself.

1. Make Friends with Your Enemy

The Huntington's doctors don't speak much about tunnel vision, but they have their own way of naming that experience. They speak of compulsive behaviors and obsessive, intrusive thoughts. They say the holes in the frontal lobes of my brain are making some important tasks more difficult: organizing, prioritizing, controlling impulses, self-awareness, initiating and ending activities.

But I think this is a fear-based way of seeing my life. The

focus is on the negative, on the loss. Battling this loss is a battle that can never be won. So instead, I try to tell my symptoms:

- I am not going to treat you like an enemy.
- I know you.
- I am you.
- You are welcome here.

Rather than treating my symptoms as an enemy invading, I try to welcome them as a friend. Making friends with enemies is about letting go of the horizon of fear so that a new, more healing horizon might emerge.

Whatever you are afraid of in yourself, address it, name it yourself, welcome it, and replace fear with compassionate curiosity.

2. Practice Laughing at Your New Friend

Fear leads us to fight, flight, or freeze. But these are not good ways to build friendships. Learning to laugh is often a better strategy.

We are taught to see the downside of our symptoms. The practice of laughing at your symptoms moves in a different direction.

Laughter creates a playful space to welcome your new friends who will accompany you in this part of your life. If I was fighting or fleeing from tunnel vision, I would not have the capacity to laugh at it. Once I decided to make friends with tunnel vision, laughing was a necessary practice. This is what I like doing with my other friends.

Tunnel vision is one funny dude. Learn to see it and respond with laughter–not with the laughter of mocking or the laughter of giving up but with the laughter of recognizing the goodness in a friend. For example, I have to use tunnel vision to complete this book. It takes lots of energy and I can't really focus on anything else. Recently, I got a phone call about my disability insurance. In a very friendly manner, the agent said that in the last months, I had not returned any paperwork and was in danger of losing my benefits unless I got the form in immediately. I explained about tunnel vision and apologized. He said I could have a month. I told him I had better do it right away, because if I waited a month, there was no way that paper would be returned. We laughed together. I hung up and started filling out the form until I got distracted along the way...

3. Unleash the Benefits of Weakness

Those of us who are losing our minds often try to hide, mask, or manage our symptoms. But they can't be hidden. To lose your mind in style, lean into weakness. Ask your new friends what they can teach you.

What practices make this weakness flourish with goodness?

Tunnel vision does not allow me to do multiple things at the same time. If multitasking is my only definition of success, I will always fail. I need a new measuring stick.

Tunnel vision allows us to deeply touch one speck of the universe. If the entire universe is present within each grain, then tunnel vision (seeing the speck) needn't come at the expense of a more expansive vision. Tunnel vision allows me to touch the whole universe by being truly present to the speck.

4. Protect Yourself and Your Family from the Downside of Your New Friends

Part of the gift of having a hereditary disease is that you can learn how previous generations lived with it. I speak not just from the perspective of someone with a disease, but also from the perspective of one who tried to be a caregiver.

My mom loved tunnel vision and this sometimes had a devastating impact on those of us around her. When she focused on something, she could tear apart anything that got in her way. Remember the story of her wanting us to rename my daughter Koila and the 25 phone calls a day?

I share this story to remind myself that if I befriend my symptoms, I need to learn to do it in a way that protects my friends and family. In other ways, befriending symptoms is about dissolving fear, not about transferring the fear to those around me. Sometimes when we are full of fear, we pass it on like a virus. Elephant dancers need to dissolve fear. My mother knew how to use tunnel vision but she did not know how to dissolve fear. Therefore, she often tried passing the fear on to my brother and me. As elephant dancers we have much to learn about the practice of dissolving fear.

Chapter 24 - Falling Mindfully

W alking my dog in the winter, I discover new ways of falling and bruising myself. Most winter mornings, Kobi and I walk five minutes down the street from our home to one of the frozen rivers that cut through our city. Kobi loves to run free-range in this unofficial off-leash park.

Now, to picture the scene, you need to realize that the disease I am facing is, in part, a movement disorder. If you haven't seen someone with Huntington's disease, you might imagine someone with full-body Parkinson's disease on steroids. Lots of erratic, involuntary movements. I'm at the beginning stages, but the nature of involuntary movements is that I cannot control or completely trust my body.

So you can imagine walking on snow and ice trying to hang on to a Golden Lab puppy is sometimes quite a funny sight. Lots of falling. Sometimes it feels like the dog and I tap dance our way down the sidewalk for the entertainment of our neighbours. I love the quiet, peaceful setting of the frozen river and a smaller audience to watch my dance.

Recently, Kobi and I were doing our morning river walk on an icy surface. There was also a light dusting of snow, making everything extra slippery.

When we got to a part of the walk with uneven ground, of course, I fell. I fell backwards on my ass, elbows, back, and head. I am not sure what I said as I was falling. I am trying to embrace falling. If I am going to enjoy life, I must figure out how to enjoy life with falling. I've wondered if falling can be like a mindfulness bell, gently calling my attention back to the incredible gift of life. On this day, I fell hard. I lay still, alone on the ice. I scanned my body. Felt alright. So I stayed on the ground. I knew I needed to make friends with the ground. Cursing it won't help me much. So I lay still on the ground and thought about the gift of life.

Just at this point, a man with a dog came down to the river and saw me. In an instant, my mindful falling was forgotten. I realized I've become that strange man who falls on the ground and doesn't get up. What's wrong with him? I was flooded with memories of Mom with Huntington's disease. Or more specifically, of people talking about my mom. "Yes. I saw her in the park and had to help her up out of a snow bank," I remember them telling me. And I started to see how they saw her: *What's wrong with her? Who sits in a snow bank? Why doesn't she have socks on? Should she be outside?* And I started to see how I saw my mom: *What's wrong with her? Why can't she remember to put proper clothes on before going out? What do the neighbours think?*

All these thoughts flooded my mind as I lay on the ground. Not wanting to be looked at the way people looked at my mom, not wanting to be looked at the way *I* looked at my mom, I jumped up from the ground.

I started to talk to myself in my mind. *Screw making friends with the ground. I look stupid. Get off the ground. Get on two feet and look normal.* I'm sure that the worst way to "look normal" is to heap shame and embarrassment on yourself and then to try to force being normal, whatever that is. However, that did not stop me from trying. I met a new neighbour, Erwin. He was very good about it. Kind in every way. This made me angry at first. Deep down, it made me embarrassed. It is hard to fall mindfully and it is even harder to fall mindfully in front of others.

Falling by Myself

In my experience, falling when no else is around is easier than falling in the presence of others. So falling by yourself is a good place to start this practice. At first when I fell, even by myself, I would get angry. I would smack the ground with my fist and curse. But now I laugh at the thought of me smacking the ground cursing. The ground did nothing wrong. In fact, no one did anything wrong. One of the things I have learned from mindful falling by myself, is that I must discard any notions:

- of blaming
- of naming wrongdoing
- of " should-ing" myself (I should have done…)
- of shaming myself
- of being embarrassed of who I am and what I am doing
- of guilting

For me, those notions lead to anger and self-hatred. I need to find ways of falling that lead to loving, not hating. If I keep practicing this kind of angry, hating fall-ing, I will *become* anger and hatred, and this will deeply scar those closest to me. I must learn a kind of mindful falling that leads to love.

An early way of working at mindful falling is to meditate on the picture of yourself falling angrily, until you begin to laugh. Laughter is the process of letting go of that part of the self that wants to hang onto the impossible, and live in a world without cause and effect.

A next step is to listen to your inner voices when you fall. Pay attention to them. Ask where they came from. Ask if you want to give those voices power over you. Stay on the ground until you can honestly say, "I do not blame the ground; I do not blame myself. Letting go of blame, I love the ground. Letting go of blame, I love myself." These words may not work for you. Find your own words. But every time you fall, use the experience to learn to love yourself. This will also do wonders for the people around you.

Falling in the Presence of Others

I find this one much harder. As a student and as a university professor, I became very good at the art of impressing others. I was deeply rewarded for this art and became addicted to it. It is that addiction that hurts me when I fall in front of someone like my kind neighbour, Erwin. I want him to like me, to affirm me. Who affirms a falling person?

As humans, we do not seem to like falling or fainting. It sometimes even traumatizes the bystanders. We do not like to see people out of control. Perhaps the falling person looks like the person is dying. Maybe our bodies reject falling as a knee-jerk safety mechanism to avoid perceived life-threatening situations.

When I fall and lie still on the ground, I know I am not in a life-threatening situation. But others don't. We know how hard it is for others to see us out of control, and so we get up as fast as we can to make it better for them.

In truth, I am just a beginner at the practice of mindful falling in the presence of others. I find it hard to picture it in my mind's eye and smile at the situation. I am not yet laughing. I have much practicing to do. I think if I can embrace falling in front of others, this will decrease fear in me and perhaps also in them. Fear calls out more fear.

But I don't know what it takes. What should I have done when my neighbour Erwin called out to see if I was OK as I lay on my ass on the frozen river? Are there ways to use this kind of falling in the presence of others as a teaching door that leads to love? I think so.

Next time I fall in the presence of others and am asked if I am OK, I hope I stay there on the ground and say, "Just practicing falling in love."

Chapter 25 - Valuing Your Life

"What is your life worth?"

This is the question an Indigenous Elder has been asking me again and again over the last several months. If the question came from a financial planner, I would know how to answer. I would know the intent behind the question. But this Elder lives in economic poverty. In my experience, the wisest Elders don't talk too much about money. He must mean something else.

Each time I reflect on the question of what is my life worth, I come up with one answer: dust, a grain of the universe. As I learn to dance with elephants, I have found that I must turn toward my fears and my mortality. In the chapter "Embracing Dustness," I reflected on Gandhi's words: "The seeker of truth must be humbler than dust." In the chapter "Replacing Fear with Love," I outlined a practice of meditating on your bones turning to dust. So my answer may be in part because I have been thinking about dust, but I believe there is more to it. For me, dust is a key to nourishment and healing.

By saying that my life is worth dust, I am not saying it has no worth. To me, dust is one of the most valuable things on this earth. Life is made from dust and returns to dust and becomes life again. How miraculous is that? Remove dust and there is no life. Life crumbles to death and death crumbles to life. For me, it is not the life or death that I find difficult. Instead, it is the process—which all of humanity is embarked on—of crumbling.

I wrote the poem below, in part to challenge my own faith tradition to take dust more seriously. I wrote this as I travelled back from a sabbatical as part of my work as a university professor. That year, I had been to Sri Lanka, Papua New Guinea, and Israel, visiting communities with some practice of healing justice. My family and I had just lived for six months on Saturna Island, a secluded island on the West coast of Canada. Rhona and the girls had travelled ahead of me back to Winnipeg. I wrote this poem on the 25 hour drive home. I knew my career and professional life would soon end, and I was mentally preparing myself and my family for the journey ahead.

On this Sacred Earth (or Going Home)

On this sacred earth
I will not curse your name
I was created for life
I was created for death
And all the crumbling in between

When I die
Don't let the crazies say I passed away
or went to some better place.
I died.
Let me go home to the earth
Where folded in silence
I can return to the dust
From which I came
Death is not some evil dominion
Where the Devil and Darth Vader mate
Death is life's consequence
Together named Very Good
In the sacred earth
Come what may

On this sacred earth
I will not curse your name
I was created for life
I was created for death
And all the crumbling in between

While I still live
Don't be swayed by fortune-sellers

Promising a better life in some other time or place
If we want to touch the sacred gift of life,
We have but one access point:
Each present moment on this sacred earth
Let me go home to the earth
Where surrounded by beauty
I can learn to love and let go
Life is not some place to escape
Where sorrow and fear dictate
Life is a sacred gift
On this sacred earth
Come what may

On this sacred earth
I will not curse your name
I was created for life
I was created for death
And all the crumbling in between

It's not the living or the dying that I fear
It's the space in between
Not living, not dying,
just hanging on
destroying all I meet
When you find me crumbling in between
Remind me to behold the flowers and sparrows
We behold these sacred beauties because they wither
and die
Behold the dying flowers; there are no other kinds.
Their withering nature is how they were created to be.

Let me go home to the earth
Where we all live in between
Let me go home to this sacred earth
This dying, living, crumbling earth
Come what may

Chapter 26 - Eating like a Buddha

❦

E ating together is one of the most sacred tasks. To share a meal is the ultimate expression of friendship and trust. In every major life event, we turn to food as the backdrop to make sense of our lives. Birthdays, weddings, funerals, anniversaries, sporting events, major holidays, romantic evenings… all incorporate eating together as part of the celebration.

It is no wonder that when working at nourishing, healing, and reconciling, we turn to food. Go to a bookstore and you can see that the cookbook section is far bigger than sections on spirituality or even business. We love our cookbooks. Perhaps because we are food. No cell in our body would exist without it.

Eating is a vital part of elephant dancing.

We all know food is important. What we can't agree on

is what is good to eat. Each cookbook claims to offer recipes for the best kind of food. A hot new diet is as common as a passing cloud. So how might elephant dancers eat in such a way that leads to nourishment and healing?

I am of two radically different minds on this.

Part I – Eat like a Fat Buddha

I love food. I look like a fat Buddha, and eating like a fat Buddha is something I can share with full integrity. Eat like you will die tomorrow. Savour everything. Eat like you are losing your mind. Now, I agree this might not be the best advice for mindfulness training, but there is something mindful about not sweating the things that will not matter in 200 years. Your weight likely won't matter. Your lunch choices this year probably won't matter a whole lot in 200 years. Our family tries to buy local and organic, but that is not easy in a Canadian prairie that's frozen more often than not. We try to avoid toxins and consume that which nourishes.

In our house, we have a tradition of "party night." We'll take any excuse to celebrate life. Party night includes nice food, drink, and sometimes inviting friends or family. We don't wait for birthdays. Party night can happen multiple times per week. During my first year in forced retirement, I decided to cook my way through a fantastic cookbook one day each week. We invited friends to join us. All they needed to do was pitch in for the grocery bill. Once a week, I served up the best meals I could muster. Great fun.

Life is richer when our basic stance is reverence, happiness, love, and nourishment. I don't know how the fat Buddha got fat. But probably not from eating a minimal diet. If your basic attitude is to celebrate, you might become, like me, a fat Buddha. It is not an accident that the fat Buddha is also called the laughing Buddha.

Part II – Eat like a Thin Buddha

This second way is more difficult. It is probably closer to the way I think I should be eating. When we see eating as mindfulness training, we must ask the question: How can we eat in such a way as to avoid toxins and to nourish and heal? I know I will not eat my way out of Huntington's disease. I also know that the healthier I am, the better it is for my family.

My daughters eat like thin Buddhas. They are a year into being vegan. This journey began for them when they fell in love with our puppy (see chapter 10). Out of respect and love for animals, they decided to become vegan. I am proud of them. I don't eat the same way they do, but I admire their deep commitment to making their eating habits consistent with their best insights on love. This is fantastic.

Our teenage twins say that Rhona and I don't stick with any diet and just jumps from one to another. There is

some truth to the claim. Here are some of the cookbooks
in our house that have survived many rounds of purging:

- *Eat Fat, Get Thin: Why the Fat We Eat Is the
  Key to Sustained Weight Loss and Vibrant
  Health* by Mark Hyman
- *The Wahl's Protocol: A Radical New Way to
  Treat All Chronic Autoimmune Conditions
  Using Paleo Principles* by Terry Wahl
- *The Four-Hour Body* by Tim Feriss
- *Practical Paleo* by Dianne Sanfilippo
- *Mediterranean Paleo Cooking* by Caitlin Weeks
  and Diane Sanfilippo.
- *Oh How She Glows Cookbook* by Anglea
- Liddon
- *I Quit Sugar Cookbook* by Sarah Wilson

Our current focus:

- *Quick and Easy Ketogenic Cooking* by Maria
- Emmerich

These books share some things in common. Decrease or
avoid sugar. Eat fats to fuel the brain and mitochondria in
the cells. Avoid processed foods. Decrease gluten, grains,
and legumes. Eat organic. If I would stick to these rules,
I would probably look more like a thin Buddha. Perhaps
I would feel and think more like a Buddha too.

So why am I of a split mind on this? First, I don't buy

into the idea that "living the good life" means living as long as I can. Second, these diets tend to be very expensive and aren't sustainable for most families. Third, these diets don't work well when eating with lots of different people. I don't expect others to cook differently for me. I want to share meals with friends and families. If we were to strictly follow these diets, it would have an impact on our relationships. Fourth, these diets are work and sometimes I just want easier options.

I need to eat like a Buddha, but I am still exploring what that means.

Chapter 27 - Developing a Family Health Plan

While we are dancing with elephants, we need to guard against turning the elephant into the main attraction. I want to dance well with Huntington's. But I also want my family to thrive. Too much focus on me or on the disease could quickly put us out of balance.

Creating a present and future family health plan has let us love rather than fear. We can plan for the life we want to live rather than wait until the last minute and respond out of fear.

Denial, waiting till the last moment, and responding out of fear was characteristic of my mother. During transitions, she would panic, and too often had to choose between bad options. When it was time to move out of her condominium and into a care home, she refused. She was unable to keep up with cleaning, cooking, or taking her medications. She also kept firing the people who were there to help her live at home independently. So we had to go through the process of getting her declared incompetent. No child wants do that to a parent. That was a deeply painful part of our journey. I remember sitting on the edge of her couch as the doctor took her through basic questions which she had no ability to answer. Time of day, day of the week, year, the Prime Minister's name, three words he had asked her to remember. At first my mom thought she was doing well, but by the end, even she realized she did not have answers. When the doctor explained to her that she would need to go to a nursing home, she had a kind of turning point, right there on the spot. "Well, then I will go and make it the best place possible." I was grateful. But some of the light in me went out that day. It was a necessary step in her care, but the step did not have to be so traumatic. I know firsthand as her care-giver that this last-minute, fear-response health plan was an awful way to live. I vowed to never do that to my loved ones.

I want to chart a different path. Some decisions will be very hard for my family to make for me. I want to be involved early so that I can use the wisdom that has come out of these mindfulness trainings for elephant dancers.

Here is what we have done as part of our Family Health Plan:

- We have created a circle of support so the weight is shared more broadly (chapter 12).
- We wrote our wills.
- We made sure the family is protected from me if/when I start making bad financial choices. Our concern was what would happen if Rhona died when I had more advanced Huntington's. I would become the beneficiary of her insurance and benefits at a time when I could make some very bad decisions. We set up Rhona's estate as the beneficiary. Then we created a spring trust to handle the money for our girls and me.
- Rhona was given power of attorney.
- Rhona got a credit card so that she has credit independent of me.
- We continue to work with a money coach (http://moneycoachescanada.ca/) and an accountant to make sure Rhona and the girls will be provided for in the future.
- We work to ensure that our home is an oasis of nourishment and healing. We try to buy organic and fair-trade. Our furniture is natural wood. We cultivate beauty and purge clutter.
- We make it a priority for me to get lots of sleep every night, even if it means walking out on house guests at 9:00 p.m.

All this elephant training is important because we need to look clear-eyed into the future and figure out how to act in love. If I am still filled with fear, I will cling to that to which I should not cling. I will make life miserable for myself and for everyone around me.

As elephant dancers, we can frame our future major issues within a mindful approach that is rooted in reverence for life, true happiness, true love, loving speech, deep listening, nourishment, and healing. That will look different for each of us. Here is how I outlined my health plan and the questions I need to consider:

- I want a happy family and therefore I am happy to take any medications as needed.
- I want our family's financial situation to be secure; therefore, I do not need to be involved in the day to day decisions. My mother wouldn't answer the phone because multiple collection agencies were after her for the credit cards she maxed out on the shopping channel buying fur coats that she never wore. I am happy to have someone else look after our finances. We have, for the first time, an accountant for taxes.
- I want our family to be healthy and happy, so when keeping up with domestic cleaning gets too complicated, we will pay others to help us. I would rather be out some money than constantly fighting over who cleans what.
- I want to keep my family and community safe. My car is just a car and does not represent my freedom. I like driving and our latest car purchase was an automatic rather than manual

so that I can keep driving safely for longer. But when is it time to stop driving?

- Out of love for my family, I do not want them to do daily care for me in the last stages. Therefore, what nursing home do I want to be in? Likely in Stage IV—typically 11-26 years from onset—I will need to be in a care home. How will we know when the time is right? How can we make that placement an act of love?
- My goal is not to live as long as possible. Therefore, at what point is it a good idea to not treat further health problems? At what point is it right to issue a no tube-feeding, do-not-resuscitate directive?

It does not sadden me to deal with these issues. I want to enjoy my life. I also want the people around me to enjoy life. So I need to address these issues from my present perspective. To me, it is freeing. When fear is not present, there is space and freedom to explore and to live. We can waste energy wishing we were living someone else's life, but the life I have is the only one I can live. I don't want to waste it. Nor do I want to harm those around me. I still have living, loving, and laughing yet to do.

Chapter 28 - Mandela Gardening

Being diagnosed with a terminal disease sharpened my vision. As a professor, I had hundreds and hundreds of books. I gave them all away, save a handful. I kept a few extraordinary books that I hoped might still provide nourishment and healing in this part of my life. One of those extraordinary books is Richard Stengel's *Mandela's Way: Fifteen Lessons on Life, Love and Courage*.

I have always felt a deep connection to Nelson Mandela. For me, simply hearing his voice and seeing him on TV were profound experiences. On February 11, 1990, I skipped school and stayed home to watch the release of the man who spent 27 years in prison and who would become South Africa's President and guide to dismantling an apartheid government.

Richard Stengel helped Nelson Mandela write his autobiography, *Long Walk to Freedom.* In the process of writing the book, Stengel and Mandela became friends. But when the research and writing of the book were done, Stengel said, "It felt like the sun going out on my life." Stengel's *New York Times* bestselling book, *Mandela's Way,* was written to share with us the wisdom, generosity, and light of Mandela. I required my Peace and Conflict Studies students to read the book when I taught a course called The Art of Peacebuilding.

One of the many things that stood out for me was Stengel's descriptions of Mandela's gardening. In the 1970's, Mandela started a garden in the Robben Island prison. In 1982, he moved to Pollsmoor Prison, where he created a rooftop vegetable garden using oil drums cut in half.

This is how Stengel describes it:

- While others were playing games, Mandela was gardening.
- He shared produce with prisoners and guards.
- He quieted his mind.
- Surrounded by death and decay, Mandela found a place to touch beauty.
- Gardening was life-affirming and creative.
- This was not a retreat but a renewal, and helped him sustain his work in service to others.

I find these images so powerful. In the midst of death, life! Out of neglect, beauty. Out of misery, happiness. Out of disregard for life, love. Out of the attempt to crush the spirit, healing and nourishment. Maybe this is why I kept the book. It shares hard-learned skills of living beauty awake even in the most difficult of settings. Mandela's gardening was not the hobby of a retired person. Rather, it was a powerful, mindfulness training ground for one who would become a beacon of love, courage, and renewal.

"You must find your own garden." These are the words Mandela speaks to Stengel. These powerful words have never left me. While still working at the university, I had helped to establish an intensive summer program called The Canadian School of Peacebuilding. People come from around the world to teach and to learn about ways to be peace in the world. In 2014, we decided that we would begin a Mandela Peace Garden at Canadian Mennonite University. For me, this was a response to Mandela's instruction to find your own garden. Using Mandela's garden at Pollsmoor Prison as our model, we found an old oil drum, cut it in half, and filled it with soil. That year at the opening program of The Canadian School of Peacebuilding, we explained how oil drums could be seen as a symbol of war, harm, and hoarding. We told the peacebuilders we needed their help to transform the symbol into one of life, love, and sharing. Each peacebuilder helped plant the seeds to begin our Mandela Peace Garden.

While I look with fondness on those times, Mandela's call to find your own garden remains strong in my ears. I wonder, how do I practice Mandela gardening now? How might elephant dancers take on some form of Mandela gardening as a mindfulness training?

What are those practices away from the world, that can deeply nourish, heal, and renew us, even in difficult circumstances, for the living and loving we have yet to do?

To answer these questions, we need to realize the difference between a hobby and a Mandela Garden.

Hobbies are a kind of retreat from the world designed primarily to benefit the doer. Mandela Gardening may be something we do apart from the world but for the purpose of renewing us for service to benefit others.

At this point, I see my writing as a kind of Mandela Gardening. While others play games, I withdraw to write. If there are fruits to my writing, they are shared with the world. Writing quiets my mind. At times, when others see only catastrophe, I can touch the beauty of life. It is life-affirming and creative. It renews me and is part of serving others.

I challenge fellow elephant dancers to find your own Mandela Garden. It can be a powerful means of nourishment, healing, and renewal. Likely, your garden will not look like a garden or even like my writing. You need to find your own version. To demonstrate how radically different Mandela gardens can look, I share with you now another practice from my past.

When I was a young adult, I was offered the opportunity

to run an organization designed to bring people of all ages and all abilities into the wild—usually by canoe, sometimes by dogsled. I jumped at the opportunity. The first group I called was L'Arche Communities in Winnipeg. I knew about L'Arche from the writings of Jean Vanier and Henri Nouwen. I read everything they wrote. L'Arche Communities are places where people with disabilities and people without visible disabilities live together in a loving, vulnerable community. I knew my staff and I needed to learn from L'Arche how to live and love well together. So we offered L'Arche the opportunity to come on a canoe trip with us. It was wonderful training in loving, living, and letting go. Each year, we did another trip with the L'Arche, which was often the highlight of our year. We were all renewed in the beauty of the wild. Those were sacred times, Mandela gardening times.

Elephant dancers, I encourage you to find your own garden. Provoke others to find their Mandela garden, by sharing about yours. If you wish you can sign up for my Elephant Dancers Facebook group at

www.jaremsawatsky.com/facebook

where you can share your practices in elephant dancing including your experiments in Mandela gardening.

Chapter 29 - Practicing Self-Compassion with Toni Bernhard

One day in Paris, Toni Bernhard got sick with what appeared to be an acute viral infection. She has never recovered. The many specialists she's consulted agree that she is sick but aren't sure what's wrong. The consensus is that the flu-like virus compromised her immune system in some way. For 22 years before she got sick, Toni was a law professor at the University of California, Davis. For six of those years, she was the law school's Dean of Students. For the past 15 years she has been mostly confined to her bed. The whole lifetime of my daughters, Toni has been sick.

Toni has been an inspiration to me. The first time she came onto my radar was about a year after I went on long-term disability. A number of friends had told me I should write about the journey, but for a year I was not interested. When I started to look around to see who was writing about living well with disease, I found Toni. She is the author of three inspiring books:

- *How to Be Sick: A Buddhist-Inspired Guide for the Chronically Ill and Their Caregivers*
- *How to Wake Up: A Buddhist-Inspired Guide to Navigating Joy and Sorrow*
- *How to Live Well with Chronic Pain and*
- *Illness: A Mindful Guide*

While there are many books filled with medical advice and many on supporting caregivers, I found few books that were written by people living well with disease. Finding Toni inspired me to write and share my own journey.

During the decade before she got sick, Toni studied and practiced Buddhist approaches to life. So she now has 25 years of experience with Buddhist practices. Spirit Rock Meditation Center has been instrumental in nourishing her. The 411-acre California retreat center has been a hub, bringing Buddhist ways to the Western world. Spirit Rock's 27 teachers include well-known Buddhist author Jack Kornfield. Among the amazing group of visiting teachers are Daniel J. Siegel, Sharon Salzberg, Tara Brach, and Rick Hanson. The center has hosted the Dalai Lama, Alice Walker, and Thich Nhat Hanh. Toni teaches through her books and by doing interviews.

Like me, she knows that a cure is not likely. Like me, she likes living and wants to do it in a compassionate and healing way. Like me, she must wrestle with how to live well through decades of chronic illness.

I knew I had much to learn from this teacher. So, out of the blue, I contacted her and asked if she would participate in a video interview. To my delight, and at no small cost to her health, she agreed.

Some teachers teach from a boat by the sea. Some from the stage. But Toni teaches from her bed. She told me, "I've received thousands of emails from people who have read my books. They say the hardest thing to do is to be compassionate toward themselves. They also say it is the one thing the books have helped them the most with."

This is a striking statement. People with chronic illness must face layers and layers of problems—financial, relational, medical, social. But amid all these waves of problems, learning self-compassion is the hardest! And learning self-compassion is possible!

"All of my books include chapters on self-compassion because to me it is the most important thing you can cultivate in life, whether you are sick or not," she said.

"I will tell a story about one of my Buddhist teachers. She was running late to get somewhere. She was in such a hurry that she knocked her drink over in her car. When that happened, she said to herself, 'You stupid, clumsy idiot. You knocked your drink over.' If I were in my car with my husband and he knocked his drink over, I would never say to him, 'You stupid, clumsy idiot, you knocked your drink over.'" Toni laughed, hardly able to get such an absurd sentence out of her mouth. Then she continued in a calmer voice, "But we say things like this to ourselves all the time."

I laughed because I understand what she is saying. I used to go into a panic when I lost my wallet. Now I just expect to lose it and am much more patient with myself. When my sister-in-law scratched both of our cars, it did not bother me. I know I will be the one damaging our cars in the future. If I want to be compassionate with myself about these things, I cannot be judgmental with others now.

Toni continued to unravel the meaning of the story. "My view, based on observation and hearing from other people, is that we judge ourselves negatively due to cultural conditioning and conditioning from those who raised us and were influential in our lives. If you had a parent who said, 'You knocked over your milk! You're so clumsy,' then you internalize that and think you are clumsy.

"When I talk about cultural conditioning, I'm talking about the kinds of ads on TV that make us feel inadequate. For the first five to six years of my illness, I blamed myself. Well, no wonder. You turn on the TV and all you see are ads: 'Join this gym and you will never get sick.' 'Eat this food and you'll be healthy forever.' So when we are struggling—either mentally or physically—we tend to blame ourselves.

"What is self-compassion? 'Compassion' has become a word—sort of like 'mindfulness'—that everyone talks about so much that it starts to lose its meaning. Compassion is nothing more than acknowledging that you are suffering, and then being kind to yourself about it instead of thinking that there is something wrong with you and blaming yourself. We face difficulties every day. It comes with being alive. Compassion simply asks you to be kind to yourself when the going gets rough."

Then she tilted her head back, thinking hard, and said, "I have yet to come up with a good reason not to be nice to yourself. Now, I know that is easy to say but I am fortunate because once I had that realization, I no longer found it hard to be nice to myself. In other words, when I mess up, I don't turn it on myself. I have friends and family who are hard on themselves all the time. But that doesn't help anyone or anything."

Some of the most profound things I have learned are simple truths that resonated with me because of who it was that said them. Hearing the philosopher and humanitarian Jean Vanier smile and say, "God loves you" resounds because he has accompanied many people with mental and physical disabilities on the roller-coaster path of becoming human. Thich Nhat Hanh saying, "Every day I walk in the kingdom of God. Watch me"—and then taking a step, smiling, resounds in me because this is the person who stepped on the battlefields of Vietnam to collect bodies while the war was still raging. This is the person who criticized his own faith tradition for being too male-centered, too focused on getting out of this world. Toni's words strike me in a bit the same way. The one who has been in bed for 15 years, not knowing if she will get better or not, says, "Self-compassion is the most important thing that we can cultivate in life." It is doubly striking, as Toni does not even believe in the self as an independent entity.

Self-compassion is not a cure to magically fix our suffering because many things in life cannot be changed. Rather, self-compassion is part of the healing path and it has the potential to free us from suffering *about* suffering.

Toni is not interested in self-compassion as an idea. It is the practice of daily self-compassion as a way to let go of mental suffering and increase well-being that interests her. I highly recommend her books for this reason: they offer concrete, everyday practices to live in a more healing way, whether you are sick or not.

In my video recording, Toni and I explore the first Noble Truth, the Buddha's teaching on impermanence, and how to face sadness. To get a free copy, sign up for my Readers Group and I will send it your way.

(www.jaremsawatsky.com/more-healing)

Chapter 30 - Last Words

One of the secrets to thriving at the art of elephant dancing is to structure each day so that you practice the steps.

Currently, this is my way of moving through the day:

Morning Schedule

- Be in awe of another day of life
- Eat like a thin Buddha
- Mindful walking and falling with the dog, being kind-ish to others
- Mandela gardening for nourishment and healing

Afternoon Schedule

- Learn something new about life
- Do a little bit of housework, laughing

- Eat like a fat Buddha – celebrate with friends and family
- Love the people around you
- Nourishing sleep

My home office is a desk in my third-floor bedroom, which overlooks a park. On the wall beside my desk is a whiteboard on which I have drawn a large five-petal flower. Each petal is one of the five mindfulness trainings, and each is a section of this book:

- Reverence for Life (Part I)—How do we continue to value life, even in the midst of a terminal disease?
- True Happiness (Part II)—Which habits can we cultivate to bring joy to ourselves and those around us?
- True Love (Part III)—How do we protect and nurture those closest to us?
- Loving Speech and Deep Listening (Part IV)— How can words and silence be used for healing on this journey?
- Nourishment and Healing (Part V)—How do we avoid toxins and consume mindfully?

These have been the inspiration for the structure and spirit of this book. Depicting them as a flower reminds me that this work of learning to dance with elephants is a work of beauty. It is my hope that many of you will take up the art of dancing with elephants and surpass my beginner's understandings of these things. My explorations in the art of dancing with elephants are yet incomplete. There is much to learn and much to unlearn. While I forget many things, these basics remain: life, happiness, love, nourishment, and healing. The greatest of these is love.

There is a story about Jesus' disciple, John, which says that in his final years, when he would speak, he would say only one word: love, love, love. Similarly, two days before Gandhi was assassinated, he said: "If I am to die by the bullet of a mad man, I must do so smiling. There must be no anger within me. God must be in my heart and on my lips." It seems to me that we elephant dancers might be inspired and tested by the following: When I die, can I do so smiling. Can there be no anger within me? Can love be in my heart and on my lips

If I am able, I will try to keep writing and sharing about a more healing way of facing life, disease, and death. But at some point, I will lose my words. It is my hope that my last word is love.

Acknowledgments

For me writing is a labour of love and one form of the art of Mandela gardening. But a lot of work goes into making my writing polished and readable for others. This is work I cannot do on my own. So I want to acknowledge, with the deep gratitude, the community of awesome people who helped make this book more than a possibility.

My friends encouraged me to write/blog my experience of facing Huntington's disease. When I first stopped working, I thought this was a bad idea and did nothing for a year. Then I began to realize the wisdom in this suggestion and I started the blog Dancing With Elephants: A Beginners Guide to Losing Your Mind

(www.jaremsawatsky.com/dancing-blog).

That blog was a springboard for this book.

To the thousands who read my blogs and those in my awesome Readers Group—your interest fueled mine. Without your engagement, I may well not have completed this book. Thank you.

To the detailed, wise, and compassionate Valerie Smith, who served as my developmental editor, thank you for making this project flow and shine.

To the meticulous and generous Dawn Raffel who served as volunteer copy editor. I am deeply honored by your gift.

To my team of proofreaders: Kerry Callan, Irene Estabrooks, Mona Lacey, Nathan Reimer, Andrew Sawatsky, Beth Sawatsky, Jamie Sawatsky, Hannah Sawatsky, Rhona Sawatsky, Craig Terlson. Thank you for letting people focus on the content of this book, rather than on my mistakes.

To the artistic and inspiring cover designer Carl at Extended Imagery, thank you for working so boldly on this project. To my sister-in-law Beth Sawatsky who patiently and creatively took the author photo.

To my articulate and brave advance team of readers, it is your generosity of spirit which enlivens this book.

To Rhona, Sara, and Koila, thank you for supporting me —in your many ways—so I could pursue my tunnel vision infused writing.

To my readers, you are the reason I wrote this book. Thank you for engaging and sharing.

Deep thanks and gratitude to each of you.

For Rhona, Koila, and Sara—I hope by learning the art of dancing with elephants I will also learn how to love you more fully. You are my joy.

A MORE HEALING WAY

Conversations on Disease, Death and the Fullness of Life

Vol 2 - How To Die Smiling Series

Searching for a More Healing Way

✦✦✦

A *MORE HEALING WAY* is a five-part audio and video series with some of the wisest teachers I've ever had the privilege to interview. We speak about how to live life in a more healing way, even when facing major challenges. I host conversations with Jon Kabat-Zinn, Patch Adams, Lucy Kalanithi, John Paul Lederach and Toni Bernhard.

I really hope you enjoy this 4-hour series. I find these videos profoundly inspirational. Links to the full videos are provided with each chapter. For those of you who like to listen on the go, you are also provided with audio only links.

In a world afraid of dying, not achieving and not succeeding, I reflect on the gift of losing my mind. In my later thirties I was diagnosed with a fatal, incurable disease called Huntington's Disease. By the age of 41 I had to "retire" from my work as a university professor in peace and conflict studies.

Having watched my mother deal poorly and die from this same hereditary disease, I set out to find a different path. Instead of trying to wish the disease away, I decided to learn to lean in, to face and to embrace the life that I am living. Knowing that my daughters could also have this disease, sets my heart's intention to find a more healing way.

So, now I am stumbling (literally) my way into learning about loving, letting go and living in the now. My book *Dancing with Elephants* shares the stories of my personal experiments and explorations in trying to live well with this disease. My book *Healing Justice* tells the stories of my visiting and trying to learn from three communities with pound healing practices.

The conversations shared in this vol –A More Healing Way- focus – not on communities or on my own experiments – but on 5 wise teachers of healing and love.

If you could go anywhere in the world to interview 5 wise teachers who could teach you about living in a more healing way – who would you interview? To whom would you turn to teach you to keep your hearts door open? To whom would you turn to teach you to expand your heart as wide as the universe?

I choose 5 of the wisest teachers I knew. Only one of them did I know before. But each of them agreed to have conversation with me on learning a more healing way to live in the face of hard times. I was deeply moved by each conversation. These are the five wise teachers I chose:

Jon Kabat-Zinn, who is the author of 10 books on mindfulness, trauma and health. He is known for mindfulness-based stress reduction (MBSR) trainings. These have helped more than 16,000 people. His MBSR trainings were designed to develop relaxation, calm self-awareness, and a reliable foundation for facing the "full catastrophe" of stress, pain, and illness—indeed, of life itself. Jon Kabat-Zinn dares me to focus on living now, rather than being paralyzed by the life we cannot live.

Patch Adams, is a medical doctor who was made famous by the hit movie starring Robin Williams. Patch has been working on building a model hospital, modelled as an ecovillage where doctors and patients live together and where the doctor and the janitor get paid the same salary. Patch estimates he has been present at more than 10,000 deathbeds. He teaches me about dying well and living well.

Lucy Kalanithi wrote the bestselling book *When Breath Becomes Air* with her 36-year-old neurosurgeon husband, Paul, as he was dying of stage IV metastatic lung cancer. Lucy, who is also a medical doctor and professor, spoke with me about true love in the face of diseases like cancer.

John Paul Lederach is the author of more than 22

books on conflict transformation, peace-building, and healing. John Paul—my former professor—and I discuss how his professional life and his faith has helped and hindered him in supporting his wife, Wendy, who has Parkinson's disease.

Toni Bernhard was a law professor at the University of California-Davis for 22 years until some fibromyalgia-like illnesses forced her to retire. Toni and I discuss the three books she has written since, including *How to Live Well with Chronic Pain and Illness*.

We recorded those conversations. And here, we share these interactions with you. Each chapter has links to the full video of the conversations. Alternatively click on the audio only link to receive the audio only file.

Chapter 1 – Conversations with Jon Kabat-Zinn on Embracing the Life We are Living

John Kabat-Zinn is internationally known for his work as a scientist, writer and mediation teacher engaged in bringing mindfulness into the mainstream of medicine and society. He is a professor emeritus of medicine. His books on mindfulness have sold almost a million copies.

Our conversation begins with Jon Kabat-Zinn, telling me why he agreed to this interview.

Conversations with Jon Kabat-Zinn (full video)
bit.ly/Ch1a-More-Healing

Conversations with Jon Kabat-Zinn (audio only)
bit.ly/Ch1b-More-Healing

Chapter 2 – Conversation with Patch Adams on Living with Deep Gratitude

Patch Adams is medical doctor, a clown and a social activist. He has devoted 30 years to changing the medical system and changing society.

Patch teaches me about dying well and living well. We explore his view that laughter, joy and creativity are an integral part of the healing process.

Conversations with Patch Adams (full video)
bit.ly/Ch2a-More-Healing

Conversations with Patch Adams (audio only)
bit.ly/Ch2b-More-Healing

Chapter 3 – Conversations with Lucy Kalanithi on Learning True Love

Lucy Kalanithi is a medical doctor and an internist at Standford University. She is a contributing author to *When Breath Becomes Air*, which chronicles her 38 year old neurosurgeon husband's journey to death by lung cancer. *When Breath Becomes Air* is a world bestseller and has been named one of the best books of the year by The New York Times.

Lucy spoke with me about true love in the face of diseases like cancer.

Conversations with Lucy Kalanithi (full video)
bit.ly/Ch3a-More-Healing

Conversations with Lucy Kalanithi (audio only)
bit.ly/Ch3b-More-Healing

Chapter 4 – Conversations with John Paul Lederach on Practicing Awe in Every Season

John Paul Lederach is a professor widely known for his work in conflict transformation. His peace work has taken him around the world to places like Columbia, the Philippines, Nepal and East and West Africa. He is an author of 22 books on peace and conflict.

In 2009, his wife Wendy was diagnosed with Parkinson's. I studied with John Paul in my Masters degree – before I or his wife were diagnosed with disease.

Conversations with John Paul Lederach (full video)
bit.ly/Ch4a-More-Healing

Conversations with <u>John Paul Lederach </u>(audio only)
bit.ly/Ch4b-More-Healing

Chapter 5 – Conversations with Toni Bernhard on Brokenness and Self-Compassion

Toni Bernhard was a law professor for 22 years until she was forced to retire due to chronic illness.

Since living with chronic illness Toni has written three books including *How to Live Well with Chronic Pain and Illness* and the book *How to Wake Up: A Buddhist-Inspired Guide to Navigating Joy and Sorrow*.

Her book *How to Be Sick* won two Nautilus Book Awards and was named one of the best books of 2010 by Spirituality and Practice.

In our conversation we explore her practices of self-compassion - especially in the midst of brokenness.

Conversations with Toni Bernhard (full video)
bit.ly/Ch5a-More-Healing

Conversations with Toni Bernhard (audio only)

http://bit.ly/Ch5b-More-Healing

HEALING JUSTICE

Stories of Wisdom and Love

Vol 3 - How To Die Smiling Series

Praise for Healing Justice

If we are to bring more peace to our planet, we need to replace punishing those who've caused harm with communications that foster compassion and healing. In this wise and beautiful book, we bear witness to how this is unfolding in highly diverse communities across the globe. Thank you, *Jarem*, for sharing these invaluable illustrations of our human potential.

-TARA BRACH, bestselling author of
Radical Acceptance

Healing Justice is essential reading for this moment in history. Through captivating real-life stories, *Jarem Sawatsky* deftly shows us that if we take the time to learn about our own humanness, justice can be transformative. In this time of reconciliation, he demonstrates how communities do not need to wait for governments to create communities rooted in healing, justice, truth and reconciliation

-SENATOR MURRAY SINCLAIR, former Chair of the Truth & Reconciliation Commission of Canada 2009-15

...reflections of a deeply curious human being who wonders if there might be better ways for all of us to behave towards each other.

- RUPERT ROSS, national bestselling author of *Return to the Teachings*

Jarem Sawatsky discovered in his brokenness a Muse and Angel that guided his life work and inspired this beautiful book. His central insight is that healing justice are two words joined together like two faces on one body. You heal yourself and your world by means of your illnesses and injustices. This is one of those books you wish everyone would read and keep and meditate on.

-THOMAS MOORE, New York Times bestselling author of *Care for the Soul*

Chapter 1 - Shatteredness and the Unshatterable

The Unbroken

There is a brokenness
Out of which comes the unbroken,
A shatteredness out of which blooms the unshatterable.
There is a sorrow
Beyond all grief which leads to joy
And a fragility
Out of which depth emerges strength.

There is a hollow space
Too vast for words
Through which we pass with each loss,
Out of whose darkness we are sanctified into being.

There is a cry deeper than all sound

Whose serrated edges cut the heart
As we break open
To the place inside which is unbreakable
And whole, while learning to sing
(Rashani 1991)

What if justice is about becoming whole while learning to sing? How do we nurture the conditions where shatteredness might bloom into the unshatterable? What imagination and support are necessary to sustain that journey into darkness, where we are sanctified into being? How do we cultivate the ability to hear the cry that is deeper than all sound and to see the unbreakable in the broken? What if justice is meant to lead to joy, to emerging strengthened out of fragility, to finding our place in the song? What if many of our basic assumptions about justice are misguided? What if a more healing kind of justice is possible? What if it already exists?

This poem so beautifully describes the transformation that can happen when we lean into our suffering and allow ourselves to break open. Only then can we find the unbreakable and whole, while learning to sing. When I was still teaching Peace and Conflict Transformation Studies at the university, I used this poem on the first day of classes to try to set the tone, direction, and color of class. Each time, some students were moved to tears because they too had experienced this grief that leads to joy. Somehow, the poem resonated with their true sense of themselves. I kept sharing it because it also kept speaking to my true self.

Brokenness, shatteredness, sorrow, and grief have been my companions since I was young. But I have also touched and tasted the joy and strength that come from fragility. My whole life I have been searching for a healing kind of justice.

In my childhood years, the brokenness came, mostly, from the turbulence of home.

Will Mom and Dad be fighting? Will they still be together? Will Mom rip open the locked door to the guest room again to get to Dad? Will Dad quit his job again before he has a new one? Often, I would fall asleep with my head under the pillow, praying for it to stop. Those were also the years of what my dad called the banning and shunning from the church community he helped start. During this time, I took refuge in my friends and my school.

In my teen years, after my parents split, my turbulence still came mostly from home and living with my mom. The questions changed. Will Mom be throwing up from her migraine? Will we need to go to the food bank again? Will Mom be telling me what an awful person I will become? Will she follow through on the suicide threats? Will I find her? Will I get Huntington's Disease, the disease eating away at my mom? Will I become my mom? In these years, I took refuge still in friends and in my excellent inner-city high school, where white people were the minority. The whole world was at that school. From early on, my belonging went beyond race, religion, and social class. But I also learned to take refuge in the wilderness, in my canoe where I learned sitting meditation, how to touch the earth, how to the listen to the stillness. I read everything I could by Henri Nouwen, Jean Vanier, and St. Francis of Assisi.

In my twenties, for some odd reason, I studied conflict and peace in university. Those were the years of falling in love, getting married, starting a family, and starting work. While at graduate school in Virginia, my love, Rhona, and I decided to start having kids, and after a few months, she was pregnant with twins! We decided to go back home where we would have more support to raise the kids. I lined up work, teaching peace and conflict studies at a university, and we returned home. In the two years that followed – which we call the dark years – our turbulence came from Rhona's dark post-partum depression combined with the sleep deprivation that comes from babies who did not like to fall asleep. Again, the questions changed. Will Rhona be depressed and unresponsive? What will I be heading into at home? Will the ringing phone be my mom telling me that I will be a bad parent? Will I get this same disease? In those years, we took refuge in our church community, our friends, and family. I read everything I could by Thich Nhat Hanh, Margaret Wheatley, and John Paul Lederach.

When our twin daughters turned three, life was so much better. We felt like we could take on more challenges! At the university, I was told that I would lose my job if I did not get a doctorate. So, we relocated to northern England for me to do doctoral studies.

I could study anything. I chose to study healing justice. During this time, our turbulence came from the death of my mom from Huntington's Disease. Rhona had another bout of depression, and as students, we had almost no money. But the turbulence also came from these ever-present questions: Will I get the same disease as my mother? Will I become like her?

Brené Brown eloquently describes how facing your brokenness can shape you in significant ways.

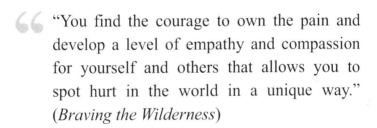 "You find the courage to own the pain and develop a level of empathy and compassion for yourself and others that allows you to spot hurt in the world in a unique way." (*Braving the Wilderness*)

This was my experience. There is a deep and profound connection between those who have suffered deeply. They feel this heart to heart connection between them. And sometimes, they unfold with each other in ways they don't feel able with others.

So, I started what would become a decade study of Healing Justice. I knew about brokenness and shattered-ness. My own bullshit detector was on high because I needed to cut through the superficial and the unwise to try to learn about healing that reaches down to your deepest sense of who you are and how you are going to be in this world. I felt like the well-being of those closest to me depended on me learning to live with this wisdom and love.

In my work and life, I kept hearing little hints that such a healing wisdom and love might already exist. I kept hearing stories from indigenous communities about 'people re-learning who they are,' about 'taking offenders onto the land,' about needing to 'return to their traditions' as part of sustaining a 'healing way of justice.' The more I listened, the more I learned that this 'alternative' voice comes, not just from indigenous communities, but also from engaged Buddhists, fringe Christian communities, and other communities.

I set out to see if I could find concrete examples of this healing justice being practiced in living communities. I wanted to see if I could show up in such a community and touch and taste this healing justice. What I was really curious about was, if one could find healing justice, would it offer sufficient breadth and depth to help address some of the dissatisfaction I was feeling with more mainline Western approaches to justice, conflict, and peace. Would it help me to face my own brokenness with healing, wisdom, and love?

For many individuals, communities, and states, justice has come to reflect the same ugliness as injustice: pain, loss of power, loss of identity, disorientation, loss of respect, becoming broken and, in the extremes, killing other people. Being 'brought to justice' is not something many seek in their lives. Sometimes, it is the very seeking of justice that leads to deep experiences of injustice.

But surely, there must be communities that model a better kind of justice rooted in healing, wisdom, and love. I set out to find them, learn from them, and share their stories.

Looking back on this decade, I really can't believe this happened. I am filled with deep gratitude that so many opened their doors and their hearts to me so that I could learn from these communities. I only visited communities when they agreed to participate, to host me, and to teach me first-hand about their practices, and to keep giving me feedback on how to share their story until they were satisfied.

My search for healing justice took me to:

- Plum Village, a Buddhist monastery and community in southern France and home to Nobel Peace Prize-nominated author, Thich Nhat Hanh;
- Hollow Water, an Aboriginal community in Canada who are leaders in Indigenous healing;
- The Iona Community, in the highlands of Scotland at the birthplace of Benedictine and Celtic Christianity;

- The Sarvodaya Movement, in Sri Lanka, where I toured some of the 10,000 villages of Awakening Through Sharing with their 80-year-old leader Dr. A. T. Ariyaratne, known as the Gandhi of Sri Lanka;
- Oasis of Peace (Wahat al-Salam – Neve Shalom), a peace village in Israel where Jews and Palestinian Arabs who are citizens of Israel live together as a model of what their countries' future could look like; and
- Bougainville, in Papua New Guinea – the site of the most violent conflict in the Pacific region since World War II, a conflict in 1988 – to a peace accord in 2001. This matrilineal society experienced a profound breaking but also was finding ways of healing unknown to most other parts of the world.

For some reason, leaders from each of these communities agreed to accept my invitation to come to Canada for a gathering on Healing Justice in July 2012. These communities so often fight to go upstream, against the current of their surroundings. I wanted to give them the opportunity to share with like-minded but differently-located communities. Who knows what might come from them sharing their stories with each other? Somehow, the Canadian government agreed to pay for the gathering, and these folks all gathered at the small Mennonite University where I worked.

Behind the scenes, Rhona and I were still dealing with the turbulence of the disease that had ravaged my mother. Halfway through this decade studying healing justice, on October 27, 2010, I was given the results of a genetic blood test that determined that I did inherit Huntington's Disease. I did not yet have symptoms, but every nine months, I would go to my neurologist to see if the symptoms had started and to see if it was time to give up my career. Two years after the gathering, I went on permanent long-term disability because the disease was active and made it too difficult to do the work I previously loved to do.

My research was unfinished. I had published an academic book with the stories of three of the communities: Hollow Water, the Iona Community, and Plum Village. Academic books are great for career advancement but not great for sharing stories and wisdom with the public. For several years, I asked the publisher for my rights back from this book so that I could share these stories in a much more accessible form, and in 2018, they agreed.

My health is not good enough to write the stories of the last three communities I visited or to share about the truly incredible experience of listening to the wise sages from these communities engaging with each other at the gathering.

From my broken hill, I want to share these stories with you. They have equipped, inspired, and trained me to enjoy the downward journey of life I am living now.

From these communities, I have learned to touch the wisdom of the poem:

There is a brokenness
A shatteredness out of which blooms the unshatterable.
There is a sorrow
Beyond all grief which leads to joy
And a fragility
Out of which depth emerges strength.

More times than I can count, I have touched the hollow space

Too vast for words
Through which we pass with each loss,
Out of whose darkness we are sanctified into being.

I have traveled the world - and made the longer journey of traveling from my head into my heart -to listen to the

cry deeper than all sound
Whose serrated edges cut the heart
As we break open
To the place inside which is unbreakable
And whole, while learning to sing

I feel spoiled. Sure, I have holes in my brain, and I am unable to hold a job, but I feel spoiled. I have had such an abundance of wise teachers and opportunities to learn to walk in a healing way.

In my book, *Dancing with Elephants,* I share about my own journey of stumbling -literally - my way into healing. In the video series, *A More Healing Way*, -available free to those on my email list (http://www.jaremsawatsky.com/healing/) – I interview 5 experts on their best advice for living in a more healing way. In this book, I share with you three of the stories of these brave, creative communities, who are living out a healing justice day-to-day.

There is more to health than the absence of disease. This is one of the key teachings of Deepak Chopra. We need not just avoid the things that lead to ill-health, but we need to cultivate the things that lead to full health. In the same way, there is more to justice than the absence of injustice.

These healing justice communities are taking increased responsibility for their own well-being. They work at personal and collective health and foster a kind of resilience that leads their whole communities to healing and love. For each community, healing justice is rooted in learning their true names, living in the present, reconnecting with the earth, and returning to wholeness even in the midst of the broken.

The search for healing justice in these pages may take a reader to some uncomfortable places. Healing justice does not neatly follow the logic, structure, or purpose of criminal justice or social justice. The search for healing justice brings the reader face to face with communities and their more collective imaginations. Moreover, these communities are faith or spirit-based communities of three different kinds. Those who value a rationalist, secular, individualist approach will likely find these stories most challenging.

These stories are not an independent, objective analysis of healing justice (as if such a thing could exist). It is my attempt to learn respectfully from three communities that practice healing justice. This is a very personal journey where the author is not absent or invisible. While I am not a member of any of these communities, I have cultivated friendships in each. As a reader will soon learn, friendship, respect, and personal journeys are very much a part of healing justice.

I tried to write this with the daring courage of Brené Brown, the blinking boldness of Malcolm Gladwell, the disquieting poetry of Maya Angelou, and the deep compassion of Thich Nhat Hanh, but my own voice kept breaking through. As part of healing justice is learning our true names, I hope you will forgive me for using my own voice.

This book is about what happens when ordinary communities confront injustice with healing, wisdom, and love. Each chapter tells the story of a different community. Some of these communities are famous – like Thich Nhat Hanh's home community - and some are relatively unknown – like Canada's Hollow Water community. Each has faced deep trauma and injustice but has found a way to respond with a kind of wisdom and love called healing justice.

The Wisdom And Love Of Pelicans

Awakened from my slumber on some high rocks of the shoreline of a wilderness island, at first, I heard a noise so loud I thought maybe a plane was crashing. As I got my bearings, I figured out there was no plane, just pelicans. Hundreds and hundreds of pelicans invaded the quiet bay where I was resting. I was in my late teens. The pelicans landed in the bay with some military order – landing line upon line – making as much noise as they could. Then they started sweeping the bay side to side. I took me a little while to figure out it was feeding time. They were working as a team to scare the fish and unsettle the waters, so they could eat. Just as it seemed to be over, another large flock of pelicans arrived. They had let the others eat first and had stay circling in the air. When the first group was running low on fish, the airborne pelicans started to land, scaring the fish back into the bay. When this wave landed, it was their turn to eat. This story seared into my mind. Pelicans love to spend time alone or in small groups, but sometimes, we need community. Some healing practices, like say eating, work better in a community. I witnessed this same behavior in pelicans three times in my lifetime, so far. The second time was a year to the day from the first. The third time was 24 years later as I was writing this book for you.

THERE IS a kind of wisdom that comes to those who sit in silence and to those who stay present to the miracle and mischief of creation.

IF THERE IS anything for humans to learn from the fishing habits of the great white pelican, it will not be found by trying to copy the pelicans' habits. The lesson is not that we should hunt in larger groups and plan our hunting raids in multiple waves. I know this is obvious as long as we are talking about pelicans. But as we turn to the communities' stories, some will be tempted to learn only by copying their habits – or worse yet – trying to force others to copy their habits. This book is not written to foster habit copying. Rather, it is written to dare the reader to be a better lover! My university students would always giggle when I told them this was the purpose of my teachings.

Some stories blow open our minds and hearts, such that we must radically re-think and re-feel what seems possible in the here and now. To me, the stories that follow belong in this group. I hope that, by sharing stories of people and communities already living a bold and wise love, you too will be dared to become a better lover, wherever that takes you.

Chapter 2 - Plum Village and the Playground of Thich Nhat Hanh

Please Call Me by My True Names

Don't say that I will depart tomorrow
even today I am still arriving.

Look deeply: every second I am arriving
to be a bud on a Spring branch
to be a tiny bird, with still-fragile wings
learning to sing in my new nest
to be a caterpillar in the heart of a flower
to be a jewel hiding itself in a stone.

I still arrive, in order to laugh and to cry
to fear and to hope.

The rhythm of my heart is the birth and death
of all that is alive.

I am the mayfly metamorphosing
on the surface of the river.
And I am the bird
that swoops down to swallow the mayfly.

I am the frog swimming happily
in the clear water of a pond.
And I am the grass-snake
that silently feeds itself on the frog.

I am the child in Uganda, all skin and bones
my legs as thin as bamboo sticks.
And I am the arms merchant
selling deadly weapons to Uganda.

I am the twelve-year-old girl
refugee on a small boat
who throws herself into the ocean
after being raped by a sea pirate.
And I am the pirate
my heart not yet capable
of seeing and loving.

I am a member of the politburo
with plenty of power in my hands.
And I am the man who has to pay

his 'debt of blood' to my people
dying slowly in a forced-labor camp.

My joy is like Spring, so warm
it makes flowers bloom all over the Earth.
My pain is like a river of tears
so vast it fills the four oceans.

Please call me by my true names
so I can hear all my cries and my laughter at once
so I can see that my joy and pain are one.

Please call me by my true names
so I can wake up
and so the door of my heart
can be left open
the door of compassion
(Hanh 1993).

In response to a rape by a sea pirate and the subsequent suicide of a twelve-year-old girl, Thich Nhat Hanh, the founder and leader of the Buddhist monastery Plum Village, became very angry and went home to meditate on what would be a just or right response. He had cultivated practices of looking deeply at the true nature of things, of using his breath to build the energy of mindfulness, of structuring life so that every step, every look, taste, and action would call him back to his true self, a self capable of deep suffering and deep joy. And so, with all these practices behind him, his anger transformed into compassion, and he wrote this poem. One could read it as an Engaged Buddhist response to 'serious crime.'

The poem does not use the language of crime nor even of justice. In fact, the language of justice is almost entirely missing from the discourse of Thich Nhat Hanh and Plum Village. David Loy, a Zen Buddhist scholar, calls this approach healing justice.

Here, we can begin to see that healing justice has a different place and focus in the life of the community than most Western forms of justice. Healing justice is about learning our true names, about seeing ourselves in the web of interconnection and change, about cultivating compassion for and in all beings and even with non-beings. Healing justice is about arriving home.

For some people, this language may seem too airy, romantic, or even naive. But this way of healing justice was born out of the suffering of the Vietnam War as part of a renewal movement within Buddhism. In 1959, when the Vietnam War started, Thich Nhat Hanh was 33 years old, and his future assistant, Sister Chan Khong, was 21. Through this brutal war that killed an estimated 5.1 million Vietnamese and over an additional 63,000 foreign troops, these two Buddhists worked in the war zones and the slums of Vietnam, searching for how to cultivate and manifest compassion, peace and what would later be called, healing justice. They saw them-selves as working for the renewal of Buddhism, what they called Engaged Buddhism.

Thich Nhat Hanh was later exiled from Vietnam because of his stand for peace and for compassion for all Viet-namese people, more specifically for his refusal to take sides. In exile, with Sister Chan Khong, he established Plum Village as a community-based in the visions and practices formed in the fire of suffering and war. Plum Village always had three goals: to model a community based on the practices of compassion and loving-kind-ness, to be a support and advocate base for the plight of people in Vietnam, to be a teaching and practice center for those who want to learn about Engaged Buddhism. Both Sister Chan Khong and Thich Nhat Hanh are well-known as key figures that helped to bring Buddhism to the West.

I hoped that, if I could convince Plum Village to partici-pate in this project, they would offer a profound example of what healing justice tastes like, looks like, and sounds like. I offer four reasons for their inclusion here. First, Buddhists are one of the longest-enduring groups in human history – over 2,500 years. By comparison, the experiments of the western criminal justice and penal justice are relatively recent. Healing justice is used by communities that draw on long wisdom traditions. Perhaps, there is something to learn about how to live together from a community that has lasted so long.

Second, Engaged Buddhism featured strongly in my review of everything written about healing justice. Being the home of one of the leaders of the Engaged Buddhism movement, Plum Village is potentially a strong example of an embodiment of that movement. Third, the leader of Plum Village is an internationally respected and renowned Buddhist peacebuilder worthy of our attention.

When Martin Luther King, Jr. nominated him for a Nobel Peace Prize, King argued that conferring the prize on him would '...remind all nations that men of good will stand ready to lead warring elements out of an abyss of hatred and destruction. It would re-awaken men to the teaching of beauty and love found in peace. It would help to revive hopes for a new order of justice and harmony.' King believed that listening to the wisdom of Thich Nhat Hanh could reawaken people to a different kind of justice. If the exploration of healing justice is to be compelling, we do well to explore what King saw as so pregnant with possibilities. Fourth, in my experience, the teaching and practices of Thich Nhat Hanh and Plum Village have the ability to transform the nature of one's imagination. As healing justice is being explored as an alternative imagination, it is natural to turn to such a community.

When the community decided I could come, they had one condition: I first come for a visit to learn how to eat, breath, and walk. No interviewing would be allowed in this first visit. To me, this was a treat, not a burden. I asked if Rhona and my 4-year-old twins could also come.

They said that was even better. So, for the first visit, the whole family came. Our daughters still remember this time.

We spent time at Plum Village before Thich Nhat Hanh's massive stroke in Nov 2014. He is still recovering and has not yet regained much speech. When we were at Plum Village, Thay was around and gave daily dharma talks.

At the outset, it is important to make a clarification on language. I have noted that the language of justice is almost absent from the vocabulary of Thich Nhat Hanh and Plum Village, nor do they use the language of healing justice. David Loy does use this language. Loy points not to Plum Village but to Tibet as a recent example of Buddhist healing justice worked out in lay society. However, David Loy is part of the movement of Engaged Buddhism, a movement championed by and some people say started by Thich Nhat Hanh. Engaged Buddhism brings together traditional meditative practices with active non-violence. It is a way of being Buddhist that engages the large issues of the contemporary world. So, if David Loy's perspective is correct, that an engaged Buddhist perspective on justice is a kind of healing justice, then by reasonable extension, we could name the kind of justice practiced at Plum Village as healing justice. But this is an extension rather than the community's own language.

When I asked them about this absence of the language of

justice, I was told that the language of justice was perhaps seen as too abstract and too loaded with connotations of judgement and punishment - neither of which they believe has a place in a more healing orientation. A monk told me that justice often misses the point of 'healing, healing not just of the individual but the society which allows the conditions to exist where people become criminals.' They used the language of healing, understanding, compassion, transformation, and being peace. They have no additional concept of justice, which is held in tension with their kind of healing and peace. Transformation and healing is the response. In fact, one nun told me that their practice is healing. A monk, who was also a medical doctor, explained this broad approach to healing at Plum Village was different from what he had learned in conventional medicine. Medicine tended to focus on fighting disease, whereas Plum Village is more focused on cultivating conditions for health. While Plum Villagers do not use the language of healing justice, they do use the language of healing to express a similar sentiment, and others close to them describe their kind of practice as healing justice.

As all their practices are healing, this story must look broadly at their practices and visions to understand their approach to healing justice. To do this adequately, it is necessary to tell the story of Plum Village without separating their vision from their practices and from the dynamics that sustain that vision and practice. For them the teaching is the practice; the practice is the teaching.

The life of the community, called Sangha, is the teaching, called Dharma. Thich Nhat Hanh calls this intersecting point 'the living Dharma.'

Rather than separating what belongs together, we will explore healing justice at Plum Village through the themes that emerged from my looking at and listening deeply to their life together.

Plum Village is a Buddhist monastery started by the Unified Buddhist Church in 1982 to replace its predecessor of Sweet Potatoes Community, begun in 1975. The Unified Buddhist Church was founded by Plum Village's spiritual leader, The Most Venerable Zen Master Thich Nhat Hanh, affectionately known as Thay, meaning teacher. Because I am trying to learn respectfully from Plum Village, I will frequently use this term to refer to their leader.

Thay was born in central Vietnam in 1926. He joined the monastery at age sixteen. During the Vietnam War, he became known within the international community for his peace work. He believed Buddhist monks could not hide or meditate in the temples when their people, who were suffering the devastation of war, needed them.

He initiated what he later called 'Engaged Buddhism', which developed the capacity for a socially engaged spirituality. One of Thay's disciples in the West describes engaged practice as having 'the potential to influence and transform certain habit energies in our society (such as materialism, militarism, and intolerance) with insight, equanimity, and compassion that are the fruits of sustained and wholehearted practice' (Hanh and Lawlor 2002,).

Thay saw himself as working for the renewal of Buddhism in Vietnam. He struggled against the conservative hierarchy and tried to refocus the Pure Land Buddhism tradition that had been popular in Vietnam for 300 years. Thay is from the Zen tradition, which predates the Pure Land tradition in Vietnam. He does not see a contradiction between these traditions. However, when the Pure Land tradition is taken to extremes, it treats the Buddha as a god and focuses on the future where this world can be escaped by entering the Pure Land. Thay's teaching is that the Pure Land can be touched in the present moment, right where you are. Quite often, he says he 'walks every day in the Pure Land.'

He teaches that the key to wellbeing is found in the midst of ill-being; happiness is not something that you need to wait for until the next life or until, through many years of suffering, you have perfected the art of meditation. For him, happiness, meditation, and healing can happen in the present moment, with each breath and each step. Moreover, he returned to the origins of the Buddha, examining what the Buddha actually said and did. From this, he is clear that the Buddha is not a god and that within every person, even the criminal and the enemy, there is a Buddha nature that can be awakened and can bloom when watered with compassion and understanding. All these views lead him to an engaged nonviolent action.

In the 1960s, Thich Nhat Hanh started a relief organization, the School of Youth Social Service, to train social workers in social change based on love, commitment, and responsibility. Upon graduation, these workers were sent to remote areas to serve the poor. While the war raged around them, these workers took on many tasks: cleaning up corpses, developing pioneer villages as models for social change, establishing resettlement centers, and creating educational programs for children and adults. Thich Nhat Hanh and a number of other monastics provided imagination and inspiration. Others, like Sister Chan Khong, provided the practical creativity of how to be present in respectful ways to those who were suffering, while cultivating the conditions of more healthy living.

Thich Nhat Hanh also founded the Van Hanh Buddhist University in Saigon and started a publishing house and a peace activist magazine. During the war, Thay refused to take sides, instead he called for peace from all parties. This was too much for the government, and in 1966, he was banned from Vietnam by both the communist and non-communist governments. He began an exile that lasted 39 years. He went to France as part of a Buddhist delegation to the Paris Peace Talks, talks that eventually resulted in accords between North Vietnam and the United States.

While in exile, Thich Nhat Hanh and Sister Chan Khong decided to make France their home base as they continued to develop their practice of Engaged Buddhism. After the war, when people were fleeing Vietnam by going out to sea in broken-down boats, Thay and Sister Chan Khong hired boats to rescue the boat people and advocated for them. Today, they continue to help to raise awareness of wrongful arrests in Vietnam. They try to give voice in the West to human rights abuses in Vietnam. Sister Chan Khong developed a network of families from Vietnam and Europe that would give monthly to the support of poor people in Vietnam. Both Thay and Sister Chan Khong visited many high-ranking politicians to ask for their assistance in encouraging the Vietnamese government to act with compassion. During the war, they tried to confront and challenge the US peace movement. That movement was so focused on how destructive the US presence was in Vietnam that they incorrectly assumed a victory of the North would help bring peace.

It is essential to understand that the practices of Plum Village were developed in the fire of war, grassroots community development, and international politics. It comes from those who picked up the bodies of corpses and buried them while soldiers from both sides were firing overhead. It comes from those who have seen the suffering of war and crimes of all kinds and believe the most fruitful social change comes through compassion and love for all living beings.

One of the nuns at Plum Village, who used to be a lawyer in the US, summed up the core of Plum Village's practice in this way: 'We do these practices so that we can see what brings us health and happiness and what doesn't. We try to train ourselves to do the things that bring health and happiness and to avoid the things that do not'. Knowing this background and this teaching, it is clear that the happiness of which they speak is not the superficial happiness so often sold as a commodity in the West. Rather, it is a deep joy of facing the depth of suffering and still being able to recognize the beauty of life, even in the eyes of an enemy.

While in France, Thay and Sister Chan Khong started a community to support their work. They called it Sweet Potato Community. When the community put on their first summer retreat in 1981, more people came than could be accommodated, so the community started to look for a new home. Plum Village began in 1982.

Plum Village started as a Vietnamese community of the followers of Thich Nhat Hanh. Over the decades, the community has grown and changed in many ways. Today, the community welcomes thousands of visitors on retreat every year from all over the world. When I was there, the community was comprised of four hamlets: Upper Hamlet housing 48 monks, Sol Ha Temple housing 14 monks, Lower Hamlet housing 31 nuns, New Hamlet housing 35 nuns. These hamlets also house the retreatants and resident lay-practitioners that number as high as 650 people at a time during the summer. Each hamlet is autonomous spiritually, financially, and organizationally, although they all share the same purpose and teachings. The community has roots in Vietnam but has had to grow to be appropriate for the environment where it has been planted. The monks and nuns come from a large variety of backgrounds: French, English, Dutch, German, American, Russian, Italian, Spanish, Vietnamese, Cambodian, Thai, and Canadian.

Within Buddhist traditions, the community blends several traditions. Key sutras are drawn from original Buddhism along with key principles of the Mahayana tradition, and these are implemented through the Zen tradition. Ordained practitioners at Plum Village belong to the 44th generation of the Lin Chi School and the 10th generation of the Liễu Quán Dharma Line.

Thich Nhat Hanh has written over 100 books covering a range of topics: guides of engaged mindful practice, renewing the teaching of Buddhism, concerning anger and Christian Buddhist dialogue. Those interested in Thich Nhat Hanh should read his autobiography *Fragrant Palm Leaves: Journals 1962-1966* and biography *A Lifetime of Peace*. Sister Chan Khong has written her own story in *Learning to Love: How I Learned and Practiced Social Change in Vietnam*.

Knowing their background is important, but it does not give an indication of what it is like for me to walk into Plum Village Community. One arrives at any of their hamlets by driving through the French hills and vineyards found between Bordeaux and Bergerac. The hamlets are old farms that have been renovated for their purposes, but driving up, I was not at first aware that one is on a farm. My first impression was the absolute beauty and quiet of the place. Each of the hamlets has been chosen and cultivated to be a place of beauty. This natural beauty of the views, the trees, and the hills is the first impression.

But it doesn't take long to realize there is something different about this place. Some monks and nuns appear with their shaved heads bare and some topped with Vietnamese conical hats made of hand-woven leaves that have the round rim and pointed top. They wear brown or grey robes.

Watching them, it does not take long before they bow to someone. The bow comes with hands pressed together almost as in prayer. They explain that, when you bow, you offer the lotus flower - your hands in this position look like a lotus flower bud - to the other person and recognize them as a Buddha-to-be. They bow to say thank you, goodbye, and hello.

Most of the people at Plum Village walk slowly, some very slowly, trying to enjoy each step and each breath. In fact, the slow pace of this life is a theme of the place. Some of them believe the pace of modern life is one of the critical barriers to cultivating compassion. It is clear that the slow, enjoyable pace is part of this place. Some of the people look very serious, which I later learn is more concentration than seriousness, but you can tell they are trying hard to slow down and take each step with intentionality. But it is never long between smiles and laughter. The guests seem more serious than the monastics or at least some of the monastics.

Going into buildings, it is clear that things are designed simply, not extravagantly. Each hamlet has a large kitchen and dining hall, an office, a few meditation halls, at least two lotus ponds, a bookstore, a large Vietnamese bell tower and, of course, accommodations for the monastics and the visitors. While the buildings are modest, it is evident great care and attention have gone into creating each place as a home. It is also clear that Thay has a very important role in this community. People speak of Thay and the 'spirit of Thay.' If he walks by, people may bow out of respect. People seem to enjoy and slow down just being in his presence. I'm not used to seeing a person held in such regard, and it creates a mixed response within me. Plum Village is a monastery and retreat center. It does not fit some of my associations with monasteries as being more rigid, cold, or stiff. This is a place of space, flexibility, suffering and joy, but the emphasis is much more on joy.

Plum Village is not limited to France. Since 1994, in addition to life at Plum Village in France, the community has established a presence in the United States. The Maple Forest Monastery was founded in 1997 in Vermont, Green Mountain Dharma Center in 1998, also in Vermont, Deer Park Monastery in 2000 in California, and Blue Cliff Monastery in New York in 2007. In addition to these communities, Plum Village claims 'more than eight hundred local Sanghas have developed in this tradition.' The community is also still very engaged in Vietnam, where they have two temples, 385 monastics, plus hundreds of social workers and teachers who are paid a modest salary from Plum Village. With the assistance of the social workers and teachers in Vietnam, Plum Village supports many projects, like building schools, wells, bridges, as well as supporting flood victims in Vietnam. All these are funded, in part, by the profits from retreats, the bookstores and other donations given to Plum Village.

Why does this all exist? The members of Plum Village see their community 'as a Buddhist 'laboratory' where they experiment with new 'medicines.' When a medicine is proven effective in our laboratory, we offer it to the world.' They see their life as a microcosm of what the world could be, so we turn now to their ways of living healing justice.

Coming Home to the Present

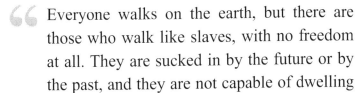 Everyone walks on the earth, but there are those who walk like slaves, with no freedom at all. They are sucked in by the future or by the past, and they are not capable of dwelling in the here and now, where life is available. If

we get caught up in our worries, our despair, our regrets about the past, and our fears of the future in our everyday lives, we are not free people. We are not capable of establishing ourselves in the here and now (Hanh 2002a).

These encouragements to walk as free people, rather than slaves, were given to inmates in the Maryland Correctional Institution at Hagerstown USA on 16 October 1999. Thay suggested you could be free even in prison because freedom doesn't depend on your external situation but rather on the ability to dwell mindfully in the present moment. The first challenge of healing and transformation then is to come home to the present.

All of life at Plum Village is designed to remind the practitioner to dwell mindfully in the present moment. The practice of **mindful breathing** is the practice of following your breath in such a way that mindful awareness is developed.

When Plum Village people practice mindful breathing, they focus their attention away from the thinking mind into the belly. The busy thinking mind is often racing, dispersed, and caught in wrong perception. They don't fight the mind on this, for it is part of them. And as they keep reminding me, in this practice, there is no violence.

The mind is acknowledged, and their focus moves to watching and enjoying their breathing. They simply recognize that attention is like a watering can - whatever you focus on will grow. So, they focus their attention on dwelling happily in the present moment.

Mindful breathing is the practice of touching nirvana, the Pure Land or the Kingdom of God, in the present moment. As breathing is the primary rhythm of life, it is here that they start cultivating mindfulness. As they breathe in, they may say, 'I know I am breathing in'; as they breathe out, they may say, 'I know I am breathing out.'

Being aware of what you are doing as you are doing it is a very simple practice, but it is not easy. Whenever they feel emotions or thoughts that carry them away from the present, they come back to the breath. The monks and nuns I spoke with reported that this is very healing. They claim breathing in and out like this just three times can be calming and relaxing.

Thay teaches his disciples that the present moment is the only moment. Within Plum Village, this does not mean some kind of existential, ahistorical, or apolitical way of being in the world. Rather, it is an insight that the way to be fully engaged in life is to be fully aware of the present moment.

The practice of mindfulness is not an escape into the self, the spirit world, or some form of emptiness. It is the practice of being here for the benefit of the whole world. So, at Plum Village, they practice mindful breathing, mindful walking, and mindful sitting. In fact, they try to be mindful in everything they do.

Plum Village is full of the **everyday habits** practiced elsewhere: waking up, getting dressed, going to the bathroom, eating, drinking, greeting others, responding to suffering, enjoying life. However, in Plum Village, every act is like a holy, sacred act where the fullness of life can be experienced in every step of every day as one lives in the present moment.

Children are looked upon as persons who already know something about being truly mindful. Children of retreatants report they enjoy coming to Plum Village because it changes the way their parents act; they are more understanding, happier, more patient. In fact, children seem to have a special place in the life of the community. When Thay gives a dharma talk, he first addresses the children. Children are part of the practice of the community. The schedule of the summer retreat seems to work against children, as it is modeled on a monastic life. The schedule demands an early start: Wake up is at 5:30 AM, sitting meditation at 6:00 AM and breakfast at 6:30 AM. With activities that go well into the evening and long periods of Noble Silence when the community is encouraged to be silent, children, especially young ones, sometimes have a difficult time. However, community and friendship are cultivated among the children. The community understands that children cannot be quiet for long periods because they are connected with the present moment. If they see a frog, they will yell, 'Frog!' Children are not constantly hushed or pushed away. The noise of children calls others to mindfulness.

Over the week that Rhona and the girls were with me at Plum Village, we noticed our children changed. They seemed to take the cues from people around them and were quicker to move into silence. We bought a mindfulness bell at Plum Village. When we had returned home, often when the house was getting noisy, one of the kids would go ring the bell. They knew we all would be silent and remember the miracle of life. Maybe it was just a power trip, but we were delighted in this practice.

For Thay, the opposite of being truly mindful in the present moment is forgetfulness. Forgetfulness is not being aware of or present to what you are doing. Inattention causes great suffering and prevents you from being able to enjoy life truly. Mindfulness, which is the basis of healing justice at Plum Village, is about enjoying the present moment.

Healing justice at Plum Village is not focused on righting a dispute in the past but is rather about learning to enjoy life in the present. It is about freeing people from being a slave to the preoccupation with past or future and about cultivating the ability to be fully present such that they can see things as they really are. Healing justice, then, is a path to joy that comes through suffering. Healing justice as arriving home in the present means it is about learning to stop running, striving, or accomplishing.

Perhaps Plum Village offers a glimpse of how a 'justice system' that is focused on coming home to the present might look.

Coming Home to the Earth

66 We should give up our personal and national interests, and think of the Earth as our true home, a home for all of us. To bring the spiritual dimension to your daily life, to your social, political and economic life – that is your practice (Hanh 2002c).

The Earth plays a special role in the community of Plum Village. The opening poem illustrates how careful listening to the Earth, in its living and dying, reveals something of the wisdom of compassion. In fact, at Plum Village, they believe that, if you are mindful, then when the wind blows through the trees, you will hear the teachings. Buddhist scriptures typically speak of four communities: monks, nuns, laymen, and laywomen. But at Plum Village, they include non-humans – the trees, the water, air, birds – as members of the community.

The teachings and life of Plum Village are full of awe and respect for all of life, human and non-human. Thay often quotes a ninth-century meditation teacher and founder of the Rinzai Zen School, Master Lin Chi (also known as Master Linji), who said, 'The miracle is not walking on water but walking on the Earth.' Walking meditation is a way of walking gently on the Earth to remember and experience this respect. Walking meditation is a way of not doing anything, except touching the Earth and touching the wonders of life. It is a way of walking mindfully, so one is aware of the miracle of life as one is taking each step. Many of the people I spoke to claim it is refreshing, transforming, and very healing. In walking meditation, when the disciples take a step, they are taught to say, 'I have arrived,' and then in the next step they say, 'I am home,' 'in the here,' 'in the now.' The goal is to bring them back home to the present moment. As Thay puts it, 'If you miss the present moment you miss your appointment with life.' I was told time and again that this sort of thing was their 'main concrete practice.' Sister Chan Khong reports that, throughout her time as a social worker and peace activist, this practice of walking meditation nourished her and continually helped to transform her anger. One nun told me that someone had asked Thich Nhat Hanh what single practice one should do to change one's life. He said walking meditation. This meditation is the practice of slowing down and experiencing life. They say, if you are not able to do that with your walking, you will not be able to do it in other ways. The practice of walking meditation is to calm the busyness of your thought and emotions and to replace that energy with the nourishment of enjoying the miracle of walking on the earth.

There seems to be something of an economic theory

behind this practice. At Plum Village, they claim we in the West have been trained to nourish ourselves on consumerism. The consumerist culture feeds our greed and craving without ever satisfying it. Moreover, much violence is created by building a consumerist culture - the violence of wars for oil, the violence of animal slaughter, the violence of child and slave labor, the violence of structural readjustment for debt. Thay teaches the American Dream of owning your own car, house and other such symbols is ecologically unsustainable. There are simply not enough resources in the earth for the whole world to use as much oil as the average American does. So, non-violence as coming home to the Earth has to be about letting go of the American Dream and replacing it with a different kind of dream. Walking meditation is one way of nourishing your spirit that is not based on a violent economy but on listening to and enjoying the earth.

At Plum Village, they have a practice called Touching the Earth. They describe it in the following terms:

> The practice of Touching the Earth is to return to the Earth, to our roots, to our ancestors, and to recognize that we are not alone but connected to a whole stream of spiritual and blood ancestors. We are their continuation and with them, will continue into the future generations. We touch the earth to let go of the idea that we are separate

and to remind us that we are the Earth and part of Life (Monks and Nuns at Plum Village 2003).

The Earth serves as teacher, memory, connector, a source of hope and healer. But the Earth is also us. They do not make a distinction between humanity and nature. One monk explained it to me like this:

 There is not a boundary between me and the world I am living in. If I don't respect what is inside, or what could be called inside, I will suffer. But if I don't respect that which could be called outside, I will suffer just as much. We are completely dependent. I need my lungs as much as I need the trees... My body is composed of 70% water. If I don't respect the water, if I poison it or contaminate the land... I poison myself. There is no difference between the blood in my veins and the water in the river. Today the water is in the river; tomorrow it is in my blood... You see when you have this understanding you can bring more justice because when we see in the correct way, we will act in the right way with more compassion and understanding.

The 'more justice' he refers to is about finding a lifestyle, not based on killing but on sustainability, on understanding of and compassion for all beings. The Earth plays a key role in this understanding. Healing justice, then, is about coming home to the Earth.

Returning to True Self

66 Dear friends, you are nothing less than a miracle. There may be times when you feel that you are worthless. But you are nothing less than a miracle (Hanh 2002a).

Again, speaking to the inmates at Maryland Correctional Institute, Thay tells them how beautiful they are. Transformation for them requires the journey from seeing the self as isolated and worthless to seeing the true self as beautiful, miraculous, and part of the ever-changing cosmos. In an essay on building Sanghas, Thich Nhat Hanh expresses the wisdom of Plum Village.

66 Your heart can grow as big as the cosmos; the growth of your heart is infinite. If your heart is like a big river, you can receive any amount of dirt. It will not affect you, and you can transform the dirt very easily... you don't practice suppressing your suffering; you practice in order for your heart to expand as big as a river (Hanh 2002b).

The role of the community, even the role of the penitentiary, should be to remind people of their true self.

IMAGINE a justice not focused on punishment or vengeance but on revealing to all parties that they are beautiful, miraculous, and fragile beings.

AS THE OPENING POEM ILLUSTRATES, it is when we learn our true names that the door to the heart can be left open.

In Plum Village, as in Buddhism more generally, the true self is not an individual or a private matter. In fact, they don't believe the self really exists in any independent state. One of the basic teachings of the Buddha is **the teaching of non-self**. The self is always dependent on many other relationships. If life is more like a web of connection, then rediscovering one's true self is rediscovering that we are part of everything, and everything is part of us.

They use this lens of the non-self to examine any phenomenon, including suffering. For example, a younger nun told me, when she first came to Plum Village, she didn't really like herself and suffered from much anger and confusion. At Plum Village, she learned that her sufferings and her joys come, in part, from those she is connected. She expressed this wisdom of non-self:

'Learning I am the continuation of my parents, of this community, it is very beautiful. But it is a daily practice; if I don't look at myself this way, I forget and go back to the old way of seeing myself.' She reported that Thich Nhat Hanh says the shortest teaching is 'This is because that is.' This is the wisdom of nonself that is sometimes called inter-being. I was told that, when we look closely at our own suffering, we see that some of it comes from our ancestors and some of it comes from the kinds of toxins we ingest from our environments, like cravings from mass media or violence from television. When you see through the lens of this wisdom of non-self, you must act with great responsibility because what you do will be passed on to those to whom you are connected.

The wisdom of non-self-connects with the Buddhist **wisdom of non-discrimination**. It is the wisdom of non-discrimination that makes peace possible. This non-discrimination is about seeing the connection between and within all things. Notions of low self-esteem, high self-esteem, inferiority, superiority, or even of equality are all seen as sickness or wrong-thinking, since they are based on the belief of an independent self. It was the wisdoms of non-self and non-discrimination that lay beneath Thay's ability to see himself as the twelve-year-old girl who had been raped, as well as the sea pirate that had raped her. In this frame, all suffering and all joy are deeply personal but not individual.

The true self is not the creation of some ideal type that is free of suffering. As the opening poem illustrates, the true self can see that the pain and the joy are one. This means, then, weaknesses in you and in others are not excluded or hidden away; rather, such conflicts become significant opportunities to learn and to be transformed. The first teaching or noble truth according to the Buddha is that there is suffering. One monk explained it to me this way:

> The first act of justice is to acknowledge your own suffering. It's an act of justice because this suffering has been denied and ignored. We can call this an act of justice that heals. It does not blame; it just acknowledges what is true.

In the true self, you cannot do violence to yourself by trying to fight or exclude negative feelings. There is no violence in the practice of mindfulness. Similarly, the true self cannot act violently toward the 'other' for the other is also part of self. However, neither can the true self simply be a passive bystander. As one nun put it, 'When I really accept who I am, it is easier to love people I find difficult to love.' Returning to the true self is about learning to transform gently and engage the world of which one is a part.

At Plum Village, every so often, a bell will ring, and everyone will stop. The function of the bell is to remind everyone to be still and know who he or she is.

When we hear the bell, we come back to ourselves and breathe, and at that point, we improve the quality of the Sangha energy. We know that our brother and sister, wherever they are, will be stopping, breathing, and coming back to themselves. They will be generating the energy of right mindfulness, the Sangha energy (Hanh 2002b).

Buddhist approaches to peace are often characterized as starting with inner peace. In the West, it is difficult to understand this because inner peace is often equated with notions of self and the individual. Indeed, Plum Village works with the inner self to engage peace in the world. Thay challenges correctional officers, saying they should have a role in reducing violence in the community, but cannot do so unless they learn to handle the violence within themselves. When Plum Village people work with exchanges between cultures and religions, they do so from the premise that 'the basic condition to have a successful exchange between different cultures is for each person to have his or her roots firmly established.' Having roots, or knowing who you are, is what makes exchange possible. The community at Plum Village is encouraged to talk every day to the five-year-old child within them. They find this is a very healing experience. So, we can see the focus on inner peace. However, it is not correct that inner peace 'leads to' outer peace. Within the true self exists both the inner and the outer. Inner peace is outer peace, and outer peace is inner peace.

Plum Village is organized around the belief that, to understand the true self, you need to be involved in a healthy teacher-disciple relationship. Thay says it was only later in his practice that he understood how important this relationship was to do the type of mindful transformation lived out in Plum Village. Many of the monks and nuns said Thay was an inspirational and sustaining force at Plum Village, although some were quick to point out that they have worked hard to make Plum Village not dependent on his physical presence.

Healing justice at Plum Village is about learning who you are, how you are connected to the world. It is learning to see the world through the lens of compassionate mindfulness, rather than through the usual lenses of blame/guilt, victim/offender, justice/injustice, them/us. Such dualisms, according to Plum Village, separate what cannot be separated. They create barriers to finding the true self and nurturing compassion.

Being Peace

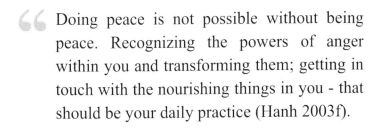 Doing peace is not possible without being peace. Recognizing the powers of anger within you and transforming them; getting in touch with the nourishing things in you - that should be your daily practice (Hanh 2003f).

Peace is a fundamental part of healing justice at Plum

Village. For them, peace is not some distant shore in the future. It is not a static end for which we strive with imperfect steps. Peace is not something that can be used to rally the troops of war. There is no path to peace. There can be no violent means to achieve this peaceful way of being. Peace is a way of being. Two of Thich Nhat Hanh's more popular books, *Peace is Every Step* and *Being Peace*, express these wisdoms that lie at the heart of the life of Plum Village.

The goal of their practice is 'to transform the suffering within ourselves and to find ways to help others to do the same' (Lawlor 2002). In Plum Village, life is structured by **The Five Mindfulness Trainings**. These are essentially guides on being peace. The trainings describe the mindfulness of transformation where each step is peace. As this is a foundational document to their way of being peace, I have quoted it here in full.

 The First Mindfulness Training

> Aware of the suffering caused by the destruction of life, I am committed to cultivating compassion and learning ways to protect the lives of people, animals, plants, and minerals. I am determined not to kill, not to let others kill, and not to support any act of killing in the world, in my thinking, and in my way of life.

The Second Mindfulness Training

Aware of suffering caused by exploitation, social injustice, stealing and oppression, I am committed to cultivating loving kindness and learning ways to work for the well-being of people, animals, plants, and minerals. I will practice generosity by sharing my time, energy and material resources with those who are in real need. I am determined not to steal and not to possess anything that should belong to others. I will respect the property of others, but I will prevent others from profiting from human suffering or the suffering of other species on Earth.

The Third Mindfulness Training

Aware of the suffering caused by sexual misconduct, I am committed to cultivating responsibility and learning ways to protect the safety and integrity of individuals, couples, families, and society. I am determined not to engage in sexual relations without love and a long-term commitment. To preserve the happiness of myself and others, I am determined to respect my commitments and the commitments of others. I will do everything in my power to protect children from sexual abuse and to prevent couples and families from being broken by sexual misconduct.

The Fourth Mindfulness Training

Aware of the suffering caused by unmindful speech and the inability to listen to others, I am committed to cultivating loving speech and deep listening in order to bring joy and happiness to others and relieve others of their suffering. Knowing that words can create happiness or suffering, I am determined to speak truthfully, with words that inspire self-confidence, joy, and hope. I will not spread news that I do not know to be certain and will not criticize or condemn things of which I am not sure. I will refrain from uttering words that can cause division or discord, or that can cause the family or the community to break. I am determined to make all efforts to reconcile and resolve all conflicts, however small.

The Fifth Mindfulness Training

Aware of the suffering caused by unmindful consumption, I am committed to cultivating good health, both physical and mental, for myself, my family and my society by practicing mindful eating, drinking and consuming. I will ingest only items that preserve peace, well-being, and joy in my body, in my consciousness and in the collective body and consciousness of my family and society. I am determined not to use alcohol or any other intoxicant or to ingest foods or other items that contain toxins, such as certain TV programmes, magazines, books, films, and conversations. I am aware that to damage my body or my consciousness with these poisons is to betray my ancestors, my parents, my society, and future generations. I will work to transform violence, fear, anger, and confusion in myself and in society by practicing a diet for myself and for society. I understand that a proper diet is crucial for self-transformation and for the transformation of society (Hanh 2007).

As will become evident in a later section on responding to harm, Plum Village strives to use these practices of being peace at every stage of responding to harms and sufferings.

Part of being peace is cultivating 'right thinking.' 'Without right thinking, we will cultivate suffering. Right thinking is reflecting the situation as it is without misperception, to be loving, to be compassionate, to be free' (Hanh 2003g). Right thinking is a way of seeing the world – through the lens of the non-self, of non-discrimination, and the wisdom of impermanence. Impermanence is the wisdom that nothing is static and that everything is flowing and changing. Wrong thinking is all the thinking that goes against this wisdom. For example, 'wrong thinking' urges you to blame the other for all difficulties. Wrong thinking is seeing conflict through the lens of the static labels of victim and offender. Such labels strip people of their ability to be peace with each step.

Justice in this context is not separate from healing or transformation. Healing justice is a way of being that is characterized by compassion, understanding, and joy. If one were to evaluate this justice, rather than measuring satisfaction or mere compliance with agreements, one would need to see if the justice experience helped all parties to be peace. Justice as being peace is different from both justice as punishment and justice as repairing harm.

Cultivating Environments of Healing

66 The quality of happiness of a human being depends on the quality of the seeds they have stored in their consciousness. We should arrange our life in such a way that the wholesome seeds can be watered every day and prevent the negative seeds from being watered. This is a very crucial practice. I don't think our society can get out of the situation of despair without this kind of practice (Hanh 2003f).

One of the central insights of Plum Village is that the

environments we live in have the potential to strengthen within us the seeds of violence and anger and the seeds of mindfulness and compassion. Only superficial and temporary healing happens when we treat the symptoms but leave the underlying roots of the problem untouched. Thay offers the following example:

 Suppose a person drinks something that gives them diarrhea, the first thing is to get them to stop drinking the things that will worsen the situation. It is the same with the seed. If you want to help heal a person, you have to help bring them out of the environment where they ingest the toxins of violence and fear (Hanh 2003f).

To tell someone to stop acting violently but to do nothing to prevent that anger from being fed is neither wise nor does it lead to healing. The environments we live in often hold the roots where we feed the seeds of anger and violence many times a day. You cannot meaningfully work at healing without changing the environment. Thay teaches, if a child gets into trouble at school for fighting, rather than blaming the child, the parent should recognize that the child's actions are a result of the environment that the parent has helped to create. The parent, even at great cost, should change the environment for the sake of the child. In the same way, Plum Village is critical of some of the Western ideas of organizing life such that the seeds of violence and craving are fed every day through media, capitalism, globalism, and some religious views.

The organizing principles behind the structure of Plum Village life reflect this need for cultivating or arranging an environment where the seeds of compassion are watered, and the seeds of violence are not watered. As Thay puts it: 'If you put yourself in such an environment, the transformation will happen without much effort' (Hanh 2002b). In fact, many of his teachings focus on choosing the right environments. He often begins with the call 'organize your life in such a way that...' The idea is that we should organize life in ways that feed compassion but not violence. At Plum Village, a number of the monastics said the schedule of life at Plum Village helped them to feed and sustain their compassion.

The schedule changes slightly according to hamlet but follows this basic pattern:

05:30 Wake-up bell
06:00 Sitting meditation
07:30 Breakfast
08:30 Dharma talk
11:30 Outdoor walking meditation
13:00 Lunch
14:00 Personal Time
15:00 Work Meditation
16:30 Mindfulness Trainings Presentations or Q and A or Tea meditation or Touching of the Earth
18:15 Dinner

20:00 Orientation or Dharma practice discussions
or festival celebrations or Beginning Anew
21:30 Sitting meditation
22:15 Bedtime

The schedule is an attempt to support the cultivation of mindfulness, awareness, healing, and transformation.

Cultivating such an environment requires creating space for getting in touch with the positive elements. Mindful breathing, smiling, resting, walking, and working are ways Plum Village tries to nurture such an environment. Such work requires a community, for it is in seeing a community dealing compassionately with the world that we also learn to be compassionate and to let go of individualism, wrong perceptions, and past harms. Cultivating healing environments then is about transforming the social, political and economic structures of life.

Pebble Meditation is a way Plum Village has tried to remind themselves and to teach others of the kind of environment they are cultivating. Thay, a monk who owns nothing, keeps four pebbles in his pocket. The pebbles are for pebble meditation, initially designed for children. In pebble meditation, each pebble symbolizes some aspect of life and identity. A pebble is picked up and held. One pebble symbolizes the flower. When the meditator holds it, she remembers the many ways she is like a flower. She breathes in and thinks, 'I see myself as a flower,' and then breathes out and thinks, 'I feel fresh,' After several breaths, she takes the next stone. This one symbolizes a mountain. She breathes in, 'I see myself as a mountain,' breathes out, 'I feel solid.' The next pebble symbolizes still water. Breathing in, she thinks, 'I feel like still water,' breathing out, 'I reflect things as they truly are.' After several breaths, she takes the last pebble, which symbolizes space, breathes in, 'I see myself as space,' breath out, 'I feel free' (Hanh 2003g). In this way, children and adults are taught about their true identity and the conditions needed in a healthy environment: beauty-freshness, solidity, true reflection, and freedom.

At Plum Village, they believe the seeds of anger and the seeds of compassion are in everyone. But they believe the seeds cannot turn on and off by themselves. The seeds respond to the environment. So, the healing justice that goes to the roots of understanding seeks to avoid environments that turn on the seeds of anger while cultivating environments that feed the seeds of compassion.

In their experience, what works in one environment is not necessarily what works in another environment.

> When we bring plants from Vietnam and plant them in the West, they do not grow the way they would in Vietnam. When we grow mustard greens in France, they grow thorns. That would never happen in Vietnam. We have to know how to adapt to our surroundings, and we have to know how to absorb the beautiful things of culture (Hanh 2003c).

Plum Village has tried to bring Buddhism to the West but has insisted it should not look like the Vietnamese Buddhism. It should be authentically rooted in its own environment. In this way, they argue that the ways of 'being peace' or healing justice cannot be based on exporting Vietnamese practices into foreign environments.

However, healing justice in this context should be less focused on episodes of harm and more focused on cultivating the environments that lead to beauty, solidity, true reflection and freedom.

Mindful Consumption – Eating Loving-kindness

> The Buddha said that nothing can survive without food. "Our joy cannot survive without food; neither can our sorrow and despair." (Hanh 2002a).

Mindful consumption is directly related to healing justice as cultivating right environments. Plum Village Community believes it is our consumption that feeds the various seeds within us. Buddhist psychology teaches there are many seeds within us, such as the seeds of violence, fear, hatred, and despair, as well as the seeds of compassion, forgiveness, and understanding. The ones that grow are the ones that are fed. We feed these seeds by what we consume. As one nun put it, 'We are what we consume.'

We consume by the way we eat, by what we see, touch, feel and think.

Take eating. Thay's book on anger begins by saying that, if you want to understand your anger, you need to think about what you are eating, in this case, literally eating. He argues that our methods of food production are very violent to animals, to the forests, and to the water. By the time these elements come to our plate, they are full of the toxins of anger and violence. That is what we are eating. By such eating, we bring a lot of toxins into our body, and we feed the seeds of violence and anger within. By such eating, we have caused a lot of suffering both around us and within us.

At Plum Village, eating is a daily act of communal cele-bration and meditation. Following the mindfulness training of non-killing, the food is vegetarian and is prepared slowly and happily, most of the time. At the beginning of each meal, they say **The Five Contem-plations.**

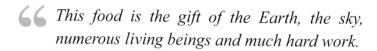 *This food is the gift of the Earth, the sky, numerous living beings and much hard work.*

May we eat with mindfulness and gratitude so as to be worthy to receive this food.

May we recognize and transform unwholesome mental formations, especially our greed.

May we take only food that nourishes us and keeps us healthy.

We accept this food so that we may nurture our sisterhood and brotherhood, build our Sangha, and nourish our ideal of serving living beings (Hanh and Monks and Nuns at Plum Village 2007).

They consume in such a way that they feed the seeds of compassion, not the seeds of violence. For them, this means eating slowly and enjoying each bite. Most meals happen in silence, or at least the first half of the meal is in silence to encourage mindful eating. Consuming is part of the practice of healing justice.

However, consuming is much more than eating. It includes everything we look at, feel, think about, smell, or touch. One example of a way of consuming is watching television. At Plum Village, they believe that much consumption of television feeds the seeds of violence. In this understanding, healing justice is about understanding the habits of consumptions that lead to violence, hatred, despair, and fear, and replacing them with habits of consumptions that lead to joy, compassion, and deeper understanding. Anyone can practice this kind of healing justice because it is not outside the habits of daily life.

Growing Roots

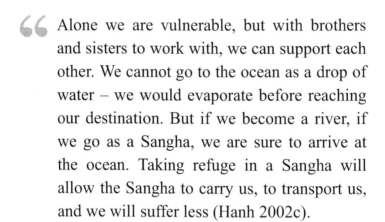 Alone we are vulnerable, but with brothers and sisters to work with, we can support each other. We cannot go to the ocean as a drop of water – we would evaporate before reaching our destination. But if we become a river, if we go as a Sangha, we are sure to arrive at the ocean. Taking refuge in a Sangha will allow the Sangha to carry us, to transport us, and we will suffer less (Hanh 2002c).

Thay is very clear it is community – the Sangha - that sustains Plum Village but also the rest of the world. Thay goes so far as to say that Sangha-building is the most important practice of our century. He sees it as the basic need of all people. Sometimes, he likens the Sangha to the soil and the person to the seed. The seed needs the soil to grow into a beautiful flower.

The Sangha is the place that develops the collective energy of mindfulness. This collective energy can embrace fears and sorrow, to offer healing, transformation, and nourishment. It is the task of the Sangha to create the kind of space and embrace that which gives its members the opportunity to transform. A Sangha should be a community of such mindfulness that just being in their presence is healing. All of my interviewees highlighted this as an important sustaining theme in their practice. They spoke of being nourished and inspired by the Sangha. Some of them said the other members of the community were like mirrors, reflecting back to them their true nature, helping them to see more deeply their paths of transformation.

The Sangha is that community that reflects 'the elements of the Buddha: the elements of loving-kindness, compassion, understanding, and non-discrimination' (Hanh 2002c). Put differently: 'The essence of a Sangha is awareness, understanding, acceptance, harmony, and love. When you do not see these in a community, it is not a true Sangha, and you should have the courage to say so' (Hanh 2002b).

The Sangha is a collection of dissimilar people with different needs but functioning together like an organism or a body where each person is needed, and there is no judgment between them When one member suffers, all suffer. When one-member experiences joy, all experience joy. When one member suffers, others, who do not have the same problems, can come and help. At Plum Village, they believe the eyes and wisdom of the Sangha are clearer than the eyes and wisdom of the individual members. The Sangha is there to offer wisdom, perspective, and insight to those who are in the midst of the disorientation of suffering. This happens, in part, by creating safe places for people to look deeply into the nature of their suffering.

The most authentic form of Sangha is created where

people live together day in and day out under the same roof and with the same economic resources. There they must learn to live together and to make decisions together. This is what Plum Village is. It is a Buddhist monastery, a Sangha, where the permanent members live in very close proximity, where together they learn to transform sufferings and enjoy life.

Plum Village people recognize there are many kinds of Sanghas beyond the particular geographic Sangha. After each meal, the monastics are taught to say a Gatha or poem acknowledging some of these other roots. They express gratitude for their parents, teachers, friends, and all living beings. Having witnessed the violence associated with the Christianization of Vietnam, Thay does not encourage people to leave their original spiritual tradition. Since he teaches that the Buddha is not a god, he encourages people to keep and to honor their original roots and to take up secondary roots with Buddhism. Honoring their original roots means examining what is the good that has been passed down in that tradition but also the suffering that has been passed down. In the case of parents, I was told how this important practice of nourishing healthy roots can lead to great healing.

All the suffering of the past generations of our ancestors is written in all our cells. By acknowledging it, recognizing it, we can bring healing and justice not only for us but also for the past generations and for the next generations because this suffering will not be transmitted anymore, but your happiness and wellbeing will be transmitted instead.

Part of growing roots and living as a Sangha is to examine your original roots for the suffering and goodness passed down to you. It is possible to nourish the goodness and to transform the suffering into happiness.

At Plum Village, they believe that, even international political relations should and can operate on the basis of being a Sangha. Thay calls on the UN to transform into a true Sangha. By this, he is speaking not of conversion to Buddhism but about the way countries and leaders relate to each other. There are ways of embracing places of suffering with the compassion of the Sangha such that space can be created for healing and transformation of relationships.

If the Sangha is the soil and each member is a seed, then the Sangha is the place where one learns to grow roots.

> The practice is, therefore, to grow some roots. The Sangha is not a place to hide in order to avoid responsibilities. The Sangha is a place to practice for the transformation and healing of self and society... In order for us to develop some roots, we need the kind of environment that can help us become rooted (Hanh 2002b).

Healing justice is about growing roots, finding belonging, learning to respond with compassion to the inevitable conflicts that arise, and being embraced by the support of a community.

Seeing the Enemy as Brother or Sister

> 66 Communicate with the people you want to serve, the people who may be criminal. You have to look upon them with the eyes of compassion. They have a lot of suffering, anger and craving and fear in them and they are to be helped. There are many ways that are nonviolent, gentle, and peaceful to help. We have many better weapons than the gun: mindfulness, gentleness, a smile, compassion (Hanh 2003g).

This was Thay's advice to correctional officers. See the 'other' not as other or as an enemy but as a brother or sister. When we 'other' or distance people, we create the conditions for violence. When we see through the eyes of compassion, we see that we are already connected as brothers and sisters. What is left is to figure out a way to respond as such.

Thay's response to the conflict between Pakistan and India is precisely along these lines. He said, '...The United Nations should tell Pakistan and India that they are friends, they are brothers. They see each other as enemies when really they are already brothers and sisters' (Hanh 2002c). Another example is Thich Nhat Hanh's 2007 visit to Vietnam, which marked his second visit after almost 40 years of exile. During that visit, he, together with Plum Village, hosted three requiem masses to work at healing the wounds of the Vietnam War. The ceremonies were to ask for healing for all those who had suffered during the war.

Some wanted them to focus only on the Vietnamese or only on the Northerners or only on the Southerners. However, Plum Village's way is to recognize that all of these are brothers and sisters already.

All were acknowledged together, something that has not happened in any official forum in the 32 years since the end of the Vietnam War.

In this way, Plum Village tries to nurture the under-standing that leads to compassion. They are convinced that the seeds of compassion, as well as the seeds of violence, are in everyone. Even the one whom we think is most evil has the seeds of goodness within. The task, then, is to help transform people by the practices of loving-kindness and compassion, so that seeds of good-ness will grow.

In Vietnam, during the war, some people threw grenades into the offices of the School of Youth and Social Service (SYSS), killing two workers. Sister Chan Khong had to write a eulogy. She chose to address directly those who had killed her friends.

>   We cannot hate you, you who have thrown grenades and killed our friends, because we know that men are not our enemies. Our only enemies are the misunderstanding, hatred, jealousy, and ignorance that lead to such acts of violence. Please allow us to remove all misunderstanding so we can work together for the happiness of the Vietnamese people. Our only aim is to help remove ignorance and illiteracy from the country of Vietnam. Social change must start in our hearts with the will to transform our own egotism, greed, and lust into understanding, love, commitment and shared responsibility for the poverty and injustice in our country (Cao 1993).

Here, it is possible to see how a victim of crime can address the perpetrators of that crime with compassion. By rejecting the need for human enemies, she can invite all on the path of social transformation.

When speaking to correction officers, Thay outlines what he sees as the tasks of corrections officers concerning offenders:

- Criminals are good people. Water the good seeds in them. Help them to get in touch with the positive elements of life.

- Help prisoners to transform by practicing loving-kindness, compassion.
- …make their life much more comfortable and joyful. Transform the prison into a place to learn and understand.
- Inmates in prison are there to be helped, not to be punished.
- See the criminal out of compassion – see them as someone you are trying to help. If you see them as your enemy, you are not doing right thinking.

Again, these quotations illustrate the basic insight that the criminals are good people who need loving help to become more joyful. A nun explained to me how her ideas of criminals had changed through the practice.

> Before I began practicing, I really saw a criminal as evil, and I didn't have understanding for the criminal. I had lots of understanding for the victim but not for the criminal. I couldn't put myself in their shoes. I couldn't understand how a person becomes like this. Through the practice, I really see that I am just as capable of doing it… I am just the same as they are. I can see the conditions that created that. It's innocent in a way. I don't want to punish. I think they shouldn't continue down this path, but I don't need to punish.

She also said that prisons should be more like retreat centers, so that those who have harmed others can rediscover who they are and how powerfully they are connected to everything else.

In these stories, healing justice is about learning to see that you and those you see as enemies are both subject to suffering and in need of compassion. Healing justice is about developing the eyes and hands of compassion so that all beings may be happy, free and living in wellbeing. In the view of Plum Village, this is not only a worthy ideal or private faith position. It is a practice that can bring about massive changes both in the inner self and in the social and economic systems of our times.

Blooming of Compassion

66 Once a practitioner can begin to understand the roots of suffering not only in himself or herself but in the parent or child, compassion blooms for perhaps the first time, and skillful means to achieve reconciliation present themselves (Lawlor 2002).

In facing the roots of suffering in ourselves and in others, compassion can bloom. Plum Village believes those who have behaved without compassion will not learn compassion from blame, punishment, and violence. They will only learn to touch the world with compassion when they have learned to be compassionate with themselves. Here, we return to our starting point, coming home to the present. Plum Village is a place where many experience coming home to the present. They believe the survival of the planet depends on such compassion and loving-kindness.

They believe that compassion, rather than violence, is the best means of self-protection. Compassion has a way of facing suffering that can be disarming and transformative. Nearly all the people I talked to spoke of coming with personal sufferings and, over time, developing compassion for themselves and all living beings.

In the context of Plum Village, healing justice does not seek some balancing of the scales of pain or merely the repair of harm. It seeks the blooming of compassion, the deep transformation of societies and persons that happens when sufferings are responded to with the eyes of compassion.

Engaging Disputes: Bathing in Mindfulness

<blockquote>
Give your anger a bath of mindfulness; you will get relief, your anger will lose some of its power (Hanh 2003f).
</blockquote>

It should be clear that Plum Village's view of healing justice is not aimed at responding to harms or disputes. Their primary focus is elsewhere. Their focus is not to wait until there are great experiences of suffering, but to move upstream to create the conditions that lead to joy rather than craving or suffering. Therefore, Plum Village tends not to deal with the kinds of conflicts dealt with in the criminal justice system. You could say their goal is to structure life in such a way that criminal justice systems are not needed. However, it is important to understand how that perspective relates to harms and disputes. Plum Village is clear that each person in the community carries within them the seeds of violence. Working at their own sufferings and living so close together in such a multicultural community, harms between people do happen. So how then does Plum Village respond to harms? Give them a bath! Harms need to be cared for, gently held like a baby, acknowledged and soaked in the waters of mindfulness of the community. Plum Village has a number of practices of engaging disputes or sufferings. All of them are forms of surrounding harm with mindfulness such that it might heal.

One basic feature of their response to harm is that they need to look deeply at the suffering to locate the causes and roots. Referring to the opening poem and the sea pirate who raped the refugee girl, one monk explained how justice involves such a search to transform the root causes. He said, 'Justice is to work in such a way as to change the conditions where the sea pirate was born, to work with the people there to change the living conditions so that they don't help to create a sea pirate.' Such a view comes from the belief that we manifest the suffering that has been given to us through our parents and relations, through our consuming, and through the socio-economic structures that feed our cravings but not our true identity.

When someone acts out, it is the task of the community to help the person and the broader community to understand what the causes are – in persons, in community, and in structures of society - that led to this behavior and then to work at transforming the causes. Sorting through this suffering is aided by meditation. I was told the story of a farmer dumping out a bag of mixed seeds and quickly sorting the seeds without any trouble because the farmer had learned how to recognize and differentiate the seeds. The practices of meditation develop the concentration, awareness, and understanding that help the community to sort through the seeds of suffering to see what is really there and what is in need of being transformed.

The second feature of their way of responding to harm is their assumption that this suffering has a reasonable explanation, which likely has some collective dimensions. Therefore, blame and focusing solely on the individual has no place within their approach. One monk explained this aversion to blame. 'When we blame or punish a person, we identify them with their sufferings, and we water the seeds of suffering within them.' Another nun explained their purpose in confronting suffering is 'to reflect love to the other rather than reflecting violence, blame. If the other acts this way because she hasn't experienced love, she needs to have that reflected to her.' The focus is on understanding and helping the person to identify, not with blame, but with their true identity.

The third feature of this approach is the focus on helping to nourish that which is positive within the person suffering. To help someone to face and transform the suffering inside of them, much attention must go to building that person in positive ways. Their practices of responding to harm have a lot to do with building people up.

It is important to note that those I interviewed saw the criminal justice system as quite misguided. It focuses on symptoms, rather than root causes, individual blame, rather than transforming persons and society, and it makes people identify with their violent acts, rather than identify with a more holistic view of themselves and life. Because incarceration is connected to blame, inflicting harm, and putting someone into an environment that will surely water the seeds of violence, it seems entirely unhelpful to those at Plum Village. They focus on helping the person and the community to understand the nature of the suffering and the nature of their goodness, so they can work to transform the root causes of suffering in persons and society, into joy.

One of the practices of the community that works at these precepts is called **Beginning Anew**. The community uses the practice every week or two, depending on the hamlet. Individuals also use it whenever they need it. The practice is to listen deeply and to look deeply and honestly at oneself and to create a new beginning in oneself and in one's relationships. Plum Village describes it as a four-part process:

1) **Flower watering** - This is a chance to share our appreciation for the other person. We may mention specific instances of when the other person said or did something that we had admired. This is an opportunity to shine light on the other's strengths and contributions to the Sangha and to encourage the growth of his or her positive qualities.

2) **Sharing regrets** - We may mention any unskillfulness in our actions, speech or thoughts for which we have not yet had an opportunity to apologize.

3) **Expressing a hurt** - We may share how we felt hurt by an interaction with another practitioner, due to his or her actions, speech or thoughts. (To express a hurt, we should first water the other person's flower by sharing two positive qualities that we have truly observed in him or her. Expressing a hurt is often performed one-on-one with another practitioner rather than in the group setting. You may ask for a third party that you both trust and respect to be present, if desired.)

4) Sharing a long-term difficulty and asking for support - At times we each have difficulties, and pain arises from our past that surfaces in the present. When we share an issue that we are dealing with we can let the people around us understand us better and offer the support that we really need (Monks and Nuns at Plum Village 2003).

Confronting is not avoided, but it is done gently. In the circle, when one member speaks, everyone else has to listen until that member is fully done speaking. The only limitation on this is that the speaker must use loving speech. If the speaker begins to attack or become aggressive, he is invited to stop and take care of his anger and to continue the process at another point. They believe this kind of care-filled confrontation can weaken the suffering in the other, even as they are being confronted. Further, confrontation at Plum Village is not an individual matter. If one is hurting, the whole community is hurting and can come and help. If one is caught in wrong desires or harmful actions, rather than blame, the whole community is asked to reflect on whether or not they too are caught in wrong desires. Knowing that harmful actions don't come out of nowhere, they ask the community to reflect on how they failed to create the conditions for happy living. Even as part of the community is suffering from harm, the rest of the community is asked to cultivate a spirit of loving kindness. When one member suffers, it is important to be surrounded by a compassionate community in which not everyone has the same problem.

Another practice, called **Shining the Light**, also reflects this double role of community as a caregiver and as co-responsible. The practice of Shining the Light is the practice of inviting people to shine light on your practice, your way of being. First, you ask a friend to shine light on you and then that person suggests five or so others to ask. This is not a practice of blaming or punishing. It is a practice of reflecting the good qualities and the weaknesses. However, the person doing the reflecting is also to ask themselves, 'How have I contributed to this person's weakness and this person's happiness'? This practice aims to transform the actions of both the asker and the asked. It is done annually over several months during the Winter Retreat as each hamlet brings together all its monks or nuns to shine the light on each monastic. So, a nun might sit in a circle with 35 other nuns and hear each of them speak of her strengths and weaknesses they had observed over the past year. Monks and nuns reported this practice helped them to feel built up and, at the same time, supported to work at transforming the suffering still inside of them.

Responding to harm is about finding ways to reduce suffering, to transform anger, to regain freedom, to increase compassion, and to transform the wider environment, so that these steps are sustained through time. Those who harm others are not blamed, punished, and sentenced to incarceration in unhealthy communities where everyone suffers from similar problems. Rather, those who harm are invited to give their anger a bath. They are invited to participate in looking deeply at the situation to learn more about how this came about and what inner and outer changes are needed. They are challenged to feed, every day, the seeds of compassion so that each person can return to one's true self. If they are sentenced, it is to a community of diverse people, who will help to care for their anger and their compassion and will examine themselves for how they contributed to this person's suffering.

What happens when someone just doesn't want to work at things or seems unable to work things out? I was told this does happen. In such cases, they try to follow the same pattern.

66 We don't blame them or force them to change. You can't change them, but you can change the conditions around them. You can ask, what are the conditions that support their living in suffering? You can also water all the positives within that person to help get them to a place where they want to transform their suffering.

The focus is still on not blaming but rather cultivating supportive conditions that water the seeds of compassion within. Another nun told me that, in such cases, they also practice 'unilateral beginning anew,' where only one party to the harm works at healing and transforming even if the other is not yet ready to work at their part.

Plum Village responds to harm by bathing the harmer and the harmed in the mindfulness of the community. This 'bathing' creates the space to understand deeply the suffering that is present, to show love to people who sometimes respond in unloving ways, and to transform the root causes of the suffering of the community and persons involved.

Barriers to Healing Justice

What would Plum Village suggest are some of the key barriers to this kind of healing justice? I will draw out five themes.

First, individualism. Individualism, they say, lies at the root of our culture and civilization and is seen as the cause of much suffering in the past century. The fruits of individualism are loneliness, the feeling of being cut off, alienation, division, the disintegration of the family, and the disintegration of society. Further, they see the high mobility associated with individualism as leaving many young people 'without roots... They wander around, not quite human beings' (Hanh 2002b).

Second, **The Five Cravings**. According to Buddhist teachings, The Five Cravings are the cravings for wealth, sex, fame and power, food and drink, and sleep. The hunger for these things leads to wrong thinking.

However, modern society has the pursuit of these cravings as the basis of its understandings of freedom, liberty, and happiness. Much of the West's economic system is structured to search after these cravings. Consumerism, escapism, and speed are some ways we feed these cravings while, at the same time, getting farther and farther away from the beauty and suffering inside ourselves and our world. In Buddhist experience, these cravings can never be satisfied and always lead to distorted perceptions. These distortions lead to forgetfulness. When we forget the best ways of living, we fall into the five cravings and are liable to drown there. Such an environment stops people from practicing right mindfulness.

Third, reliance on fear and violence. In too many societies, violence is seen as a tool through which one can build safety and suppress unwanted violence. However, Thay sees violence as the inability to look with compassion. It cannot create safety because it does nothing to make the other feel safe. It cannot be used as a tool to suppress unwanted violence because violence cannot be suppressed. They also believe that seeking after cravings create all kinds of violence in the world. Fear for security and for protecting that which has been acquired through craving also increases violence. Violence, however it is used, feeds the seeds of violence, despair, and hatred. Feeding those seeds acts as a barrier to being peace.

Fourth, **habit-energy**. Habit-energy is the old patterns, patterns of rushing, patterns of responding out of violence or fear, patterns of judging. Habit-energy pulls us back to the old ways of doing things. These ways can be transformed through acknowledging them and speaking to them. But without engaging the old patterns or habit-energy, it is not possible to create the response of mindful living.

Fifth, **wrong perception/wrong thinking**. It is wrong thinking that 'makes you hateful, angry, suffering in self, and makes others suffer' (Hanh 2003g). Wrong thinking is thinking that distorts reality. It is the thinking that flows from not following the wisdoms of non-self, non-discrimination, and impermanence. Guilt and blame are two examples of wrong perception that perpetuate violence.

Final Words

Plum Village offers the story of a community whose approach to healing justice was born out of their experience of the worst kinds of crime and violence and the structural injustices of intra-national and international political self-interest. Drawing on a 2500-year tradition of Buddhism, their understanding of healing justice is rooted in compassion, understanding, and loving-kindness at every step of the process.

For them, healing justice is about learning to look deeply into the nature of suffering to find the path to well-being. The well-being of which they speak is not so much focused on responding to injustice or repairing harm. Rather, it is about learning one's true names, or as the opening poem puts it, 'to see that my joy and pain are one… so I can wake up and so the door of my heart can be left open, the door of compassion.'

At Plum Village, they believe that such compassionate transformation is available to all beings and that all beings on our planets are now dependent on humans rediscovering such ways as the basis for our ecological, sociological, and economical ways of being.

Chapter 3- Hollow Water Community and The Holistic Circle Healing

T he sun peaks over the horizon, and a thick fog clings about five feet above the ground. As I drive the two hours north of Winnipeg towards Hollow Water, I enter through gates of golden aspens and evergreens. It's an early October morning, and the fall of 2006 is in full color. I know that I come at a time of a change of seasons, not just for the land, but also for the community of Hollow Water that I am going to meet.

Hollow Water commonly refers to the four neighboring communities of Manigotagan, Ahbaming, Seymourville, and Hollow Water First Nation in central Manitoba, Canada. Hollow Water First Nation is an Anishinabe or Ojibway community. The other three communities are Métis communities. Together, the four communities total about one thousand people.

In significant parts of the restorative justice movement,

Hollow Water has become almost a mythic story, a story of inspiration to many. Today, Hollow Water is seen as 'the most mature and well-accepted of any healing program in Canada.'

This particular story has grabbed attention for many reasons. First, Hollow Water faced a depth of harm and destruction, which startled human sensibility and disturbed the stereotypes of friendly Canadian living. In the 1980s, the community was reported to have an alcohol abuse rate of nearly 100%, unemployment over 70%, and there was a severe shortage of appropriate housing. As they started to work at community healing, they discovered that alcohol abuse and unemployment covered other abuses hidden in the dark corners of Hollow Water, particularly sexual violence. **The community had chronic sexual abuse problems going back three generations, and estimates were that 66%-80% of the population had been victims of sexual abuse and 35-50% of the population had been victimizers.** These harms covered the whole range of sexual abuse. Not just men had victimized others but so had women, children, Elders, parents, and extended family members. All of the victimizers had previously been victims. During this time, the community rated its own community health at 0 (having no health or wellness) on a scale of 0-10. Hollow Water was a broken community.

But international attention and inspiration do not come from brokenness alone. In the 1980s, Hollow Water and the surrounding communities initiated a healing movement to respond to this brokenness. As sexual abuse lay at the root of many problems, not least of which was harmful to children, sexual abuse would, in the beginning, become the focus of a healing movement. Over time, the community developed a new partnership with the Western systems of justice and social service based on the needs of the community, a partnership called **Community Holistic Circle Healing** or CHCH.

Hollow Water rejected incarceration as the primary mode of dealing with sexual abuse and sought to keep victims and victimizers in the community and to support them on a healing path. To do this, they began the long road of returning to some of the traditional teachings and ceremonies. They also developed a **13-step process and protocol for responding to sexual abuse disclosures.** Eventually, researchers, government officials, and other Aboriginal communities started to notice what was happening. In 2001, after several positive studies, the government commissioned an economic analysis of Hollow Water that showed, in their practice of working at sexual abuse through healing forms of justice, only two out of 107 victimizers were found to have re-offended, a reoffending rate more than six times lower than the national average rate for sexual abusing. The economic analysis also concluded that, for every two dollars the provincial and federal governments spent on this local healing practice, they received at least $6.21-$15.90 worth of services.

I was driving toward a legend. When I decided to learn

about healing justice from communities, I expected that I would need to visit Hollow Water. This was confirmed when I read everything written about healing justice. Aboriginal communities of Canada were featured as among the leaders of this movement. Rupert Ross and the journal produced by the Native Law Centre of Canada at the University of *Saskatchewan, Justice as Healing,* were presented as two significant catalysts in the Aboriginal healing justice movement. Both sources used Hollow Water as one of their key examples of justice as healing. I had to go to Hollow Water.

Not having had previous contact with the community, I reached out to them and explained my motivation for wanting to come learn from them. The CHCH workers, Board, and Elders work by consensus, and so my request had to be approved by a wide circle of community members. They did not bother much with my CV or academic background. They wanted to know why I wanted to learn, what I would do with the information, and if they would have space to tell their own story. Most of all, I think they wanted to get a sense of who I was and to see if they could trust me. Indigenous people have hard-earned reasons not to trust white Christians from universities. But I knew that, if they did not trust me, I would not learn what I needed to learn. Eventually, I got word that I could come.

As I drove into the community, I came with some fear and trembling. I knew I would be walking next to those whose ability to find healing in the midst of brokenness had inspired people from around the world. I knew I would be walking next to victims of sexual abuse and next to their victimizers. I was going into a culture for which I had deep respect, but which was very different from my own. Would it be possible for me to learn the touch and taste of healing justice?

What I discovered when I arrived in Hollow Water was quite different from what I had read in the books and studies. The Community Holistic Circle Healing organization and the healing momentum in the community were at a low point. In some ways, the healing movement had been declining over eight years. Just as I arrived, CHCH staff together with representatives of the community were beginning to examine what had happened and to re-envision what could happen with healing at Hollow Water. In my interviews, hardly anyone mentioned the 13-step process that had inspired the world. As I listened to workers and community members, many of whom had twenty years of experience in the ups and downs of healing, I learned the story and practices of Hollow Water were not confined to sexual abuse or processes to decrease reoffending. Even while some vital outward signs of health were in decline, a much broader and deeper vision of healing justice was emerging. This vision was not based on naïve idealism but was rooted in the experience of a twenty-year path of working at and, sometimes, failing at, holistic healing across the whole community.

Phase 1: We Had Everything We Needed To Live And Be Connected To Creator (Creation-1860s)

66 At the time of contact, we had our own
   structures, healing, and language. We had
   everything that we needed to live and be
   connected to Creator.

Elder at Hollow Water

So begins the story of Hollow Water in 1984 when a group started to meet to talk about what they could do to support healing in their community. That group used whatever they could find that might help, turning first to healing in themselves and finding support from Western therapy models. However, they eventually discovered that healing, for them, meant recovering a traditional path. This meant trying to learn what life was like before the abuse took hold and before colonialism disrupted life in Hollow Water. To understand what Hollow Water is up to now, we must go back to the beginning, to Creator and to creation.

Their memories of those pre-colonial times are sketchy. Colonialism actively interrupted handing down of traditions. Hollow Water is working to bring back their traditions by engaging Elders from inside and outside of their community to come and help them learn their traditions again. They also sponsored learning projects, like a research project into the clan structure, to recover whatever they can about how life had once been organized.

Their goal is not to return to some golden age of perfection. Several people told me they do not think life was perfect before colonialism. People have always harmed others, but before colonialism, there were ways of structuring life that made harm less likely, and there were ways to heal from conflicts as they arose. They want to recover this structuring of life.

One Elder put it this way:

> Some time ago we didn't need to have jails, police, mental institutions... all the things that are currently out there that we have to go to for help. We didn't have those things before. We didn't need them. We have to get back to that way of living, that way of being again so that we don't need those systems.

Those at CHCH seem to believe **healing is about a community returning to their former way of living in which justice and social service systems were no longer needed.**

The language of justice does not seem to figure strongly at Hollow Water. They speak of holistic community healing and sometimes wellness. They talk about respect and truthfulness and other virtues. I asked one Elder about this lack of focus on justice, and he said the whole traditional system working together is justice. Another said their way of healing is their way of justice. What is clear is that they do not have some prior concept of justice as punishment or justice as anything that is later balanced against or held in tension with other virtues. To understand what healing justice is at Hollow Water, it is necessary to understand their pre-colonial vision and practices.

As best as I can understand the traditional vision of healing justice, that teaching includes a few key dynamics:

- Embodying the Seven Sacred Teachings and 'Living a Good Life;'
- Recognizing you are the land; and
- Interconnecting and balancing.

Embodying the Seven Sacred Teachings and Living a Good Life

Hollow Water is significant because it is rooted in the Anishinabe way of being. As Burma Bushie, one of the original leaders of CHCH, says, 'The Spirit piece is at the very core.' **The Seven Sacred Teachings** were given by Creator and handed down through the generations by the Elders. These teachings form the seedbed for healing in Hollow Water. The Seven Sacred Teachings of the Anishinabe include: courage; spiritual knowledge; respect for others, the earth, and for oneself; honesty;

humility; love and truth. An Elder told me they form the basis, not just of how to relate to each other, but also to Creator, to the land, and to social structures.

These teachings are the law of the Anishinabe. They are not primarily prohibitions against certain behaviors. They are teachings about how to attain what they called **p'mad'ziwin, translated Living the Good Life**. Hallowell, an American anthropologist, describes p'mad'ziwin as '…life in the fullest sense, life in the sense of health, longevity, and well-being, not only for oneself but for one's family. The goal of living was a good life, and the Good Life involved p'mad'ziwin'. Living the Good Life is expressed by the community in a related concept called w'daeb'awaewe, 'the truth as we know it.' Couture claims these two concepts are Hollow Water's guiding core energy. My time listening at Hollow Water confirms this sense. When asked how to explain healing in Hollow Water to outsiders, one CHCH worker said, 'Healing is living.' Numerous respondents said healing was about learning to be Anishinabe.

Recognizing You Are the Land

Creation, meaning the land, the animals, and all the many interdependent relationships within it, is central to understanding the Anishinabe approach to life and healing. This theme surfaced in every person who shared their stories with me. For them, healing justice is not possible without the right kind of relationship with creation. They are clear that humans do not live above creation. They are creation. Some even suggested that trying to live above or be stronger than something else is the root of abuse. For them, change toward healing comes from staying close to creation. They realize they are dependent on it. One Elder gave me this explanation:

> **Once you recognize that as a human being you are the air, the water, the plant life and the animal life, and we take this in to sustain your physical nature, once you can see that, understand that, recognize that, I think you are on a good road of learning and becoming complete and being on a healing way.**

Other research on the Anishinabe supports this primary role of creation within the Hollow Water approach to healing. In describing the Anishinabe worldview, Sivell-Ferri says they see creation as Creator's gift of beauty and mystery in which humans are the last and most dependent of all creatures. Many of the Anishinabe practices of healing, such as sweat lodge ceremonies, smudging ceremonies and prayers, come out of these teachings of the connections within creation.

Cultivating Interconnection and Wholeness

Healing justice flows out of this understanding of creation and of living the Good Life; therefore, it follows the laws of interconnectedness and wholeness. For those at Hollow Water, healing is about learning how you are connected to yourself, your family, your extended family, your community, your Elders, strangers, and the land. All of these are from Creator and as a person at Hollow Water quipped, 'Creator don't make no junk.' Their way of justice works on the imagination of connection. Western methods, like incarceration, work on the imagination of disconnection. For those at Hollow Water, prisons only remove people from what they need to heal – the land, the community, the Good Life. Their focus on connection is a double focus. On one hand, abuse can be understood as painful experiences passed down through the generations; therefore, to heal it is important to understand the kinds of abuse present in your family tree. On the other hand, interconnection is about learning about good and healthy connection. It is about learning to see the gift and beauty of each person and how each is needed by all the rest. Healing expands positive interconnections and creates a holistic community, which has members who know who they are, and which is compassionately connected to all of creation.

Recovering Pre-Colonial Practices

As I understand the traditional vision of healing at Hollow Water, it is embedded in the traditional practices that structured day-to-day life, in particular in the lodges, ceremonies, and the clan system.

Ceremony structured the life and imagination of the Anishinabe in pre-colonial times. One elder told me there was a song for everything, from the daily task of cutting down trees to the special gatherings of a particular ceremony. **All of life was ceremony.** When asked if these songs were part of justice practices, the Elder immediately agreed. 'Creator is the one who gave us everything. So anytime we use anything on the land we have to acknowledge Creator for the gift.' Acknowledging Creator seems to be a significant function of much of the ceremony. When I went out with several women of Hollow Water to pick medicine from the river, there were ceremonies an Elder had to perform before we set out and prayers given through tobacco offerings as we picked. They do not see these prayers as magic but as acknowledging Creator. They seem to believe that, when we stop acknowledging Creator, negative things start to happen and healing decreases.

Similarly, there are multiple lodges set up in different places for ceremony and for teaching the people the best ways to survive together. These are **The Sweat Lodge, The Moon lodge, and The Midewin Lodge** to name a few. These lodges, in their very structure and organization, teach about how to live a full life of respect. The Elders are responsible for explaining to people when they are ready, the meanings of the lodges.

One story that I was told regarding **The Moon Lodge** was that, traditionally, women were held in great respect because they were the only ones who could carry life within them. When women live in the bush in close quarters, their menstrual cycles (called their Moon Time) tend to get synchronized. So, when their Moon Time was coming, the women would go to the Moon Lodge. This was a place off in the bush where they would live apart from the men. There would be ceremonies done at these lodges to give thanks to Grandmother Moon and to Creator for the gifts of life. When the moon time was over, the women would return. Some would be pregnant, others not. The men believed the ceremony made them pregnant. Accordingly, the women were held in sacred esteem. When science taught them that the sperm, not the ceremony, made the women pregnant, women became more like objects. Creator was not needed. Respect and sacred esteem vanished. Women and children were abused. Of course, there were many other factors involved in the rise of abuse, but those at Hollow Water have learned through the worst kind of experience that not acknowledging Creator for the gift of life has dire and often unintended consequences. The ceremonies and lodges teach them how to live a life of respect and acknowledgment for all the sacred gifts of Creator.

Before colonization, the Anishinabe relied on the clan system as a way of organizing life, so each person was cared for and had clear responsibilities to care for others. I was told multiple times that, when you are assigned a clan, the clan represents a responsibility to yourself, to the community, and to the world. Families are not necessarily all in the same clan, so the clan system has a cross-stitching effect of connecting various sections of the community with a responsibility to work together for the benefit of the whole. An Elder explained the purpose of the clan system to me.

66 In the clan system, each specific clan has a responsibility. Each person has a clan and each family has a kinship base, gender and family roots. You all know what that responsibility is. Along with knowing your clan and your responsibility you are also taught the Good Life. That's a lodge we don't have a home for yet - the Mindowin lodge. In that lodge, you are given teaching on the good life, how to live the good life, and how you are connected to the rivers, to the wind, and to all elements. All that is explained in the making of the lodge. And everything in the lodge is significant for living the good life. If you follow that way and if you follow the clan responsibility, you learn the teaching of the law. Those are the basis of what keeps you centered and grounded in your walking... That means everything that you do is vital in living the good life, not just responding to abuse... You grew up, and you knew exactly what to expect if you didn't follow. If you harmed someone it was not only harming him, but yourself and your whole clan... If you hurt

someone from another clan, your whole clan is responsible.

In this first phase of pre-colonial contact, Hollow Water Community had visions and practices of traditional law, which led to but also embodied the Good Life.

Phase 2: 'We Lost Everything Over The Last 130-140 Years' (1860s-Continuing)

> The ceremonies which were always there and always used for well-being were put aside by an external system that saw that this is what maintains these people. Our people were seen as being in the way of progress. As long as we maintained that the land is sacred, the resources of Mother Earth are sacred, that they need to be protected and used sustainably and responsibly, we were seen as being in the way. And that was the main idea of colonialization – a breakdown of a system that protected the people and the source of life... so that capitalism could gain momentum.

That is how one Elder explained colonialism to me. Many others also have come to see that the forces of colonialization and assimilation lay behind the extraordinarily high rates of abuse.

The many systems that were supposed to be helping the community - the justice system, social service system, education system, and the churches - were actually failing them. The arrival of these systems caused far-reaching loss of cultural values. Here are some of these losses:

- language in which is embedded the sacred teachings and the imagination of how to survive together
- connection to land, which taught them about Creator and about how to structure life together
- traditional ceremonies and ways of healing and cleansing
- transfer of parenting and survival skills (which was broken by the residential school system)
- relationships between Elders and youth
- respected place traditionally given to women
- traditional governance traditions as the Indian Act forcibly sidelined traditional leadership for new short-term elected leadership
- worldview and relationship with Creator
- knowledge of how to respond to conflicts, as justice and social services and churches tried to take control of community problems
- economic well-being
- traditional employment
- sense of identity
- awareness of the sacredness of life.

These losses of the sacredness of life found expression in a most unsacred way - sexual abuse of women and children, the very symbols of sacred life. The sexual abuse epidemic in Hollow Water began with colonialism. Colonialism destroyed the social order and traditional mechanisms that taught a practice of a life based on sacred respect. Other effects of these losses were family violence, alcoholism, oppression of each other, and internalized violence.

In the 130 years of the second phase, the Hollow Water community lost everything through the attempts of assimilation and attempts at helping that come from various parts of the Western communities.

Phase 3: Hitting Bottom And Initiating Healing (1984-1993)

In 1984, a group later named the Resource Team started to meet to see how they could support community healing. The group consisted of about 24 people, mostly women, and included representatives of many of the service sectors of the community: Native Drug and Alcohol Program, Welfare Administrator, Child and Family Services Director, community volunteers, Catholic and Mennonite church representatives, chief and council, mayors, school representatives. The group was open to anyone and met every two weeks. Their focus was to create a healthy community. Significantly, the initial focus was not sexual abuse. They looked at alcohol abuse and many issues to do with their youth. They could see complex problems in the young people, and they tried to find ways to intervene and support.

They quickly learned the first step was to work at healing for themselves. Most of the members were alcoholics. They knew they had to be on a healing journey if they were to assist in the community healing. A core group went to the **New Direction Training at the Alkali Lake Community**. Eventually, this group and others in the community started to understand that part of the roots of their alcoholism and the problems the young people were experiencing was rooted in sexual abuse. They hosted a community workshop entitled 'Nutrition and Health.' At this workshop, a survey revealed that nine out of ten people in attendance had been sexually abused or had abused others or both. The group started to see the attention to sexual abuse as the necessary beginning to reclaiming community ownership of their problems and the broader issues of community health.

Around this time, a young girl disclosed that an uncle had molested her. The uncle went to jail, and the girl began a long road of drinking and drugs. Many wondered how this kind of justice served the girl, the uncle, or the community. The community decided they could no longer sit by and watch what the system was doing to their community. However, they needed help.

In 1989, they organized a two-year training course on sexual abuse and recruited people from each of the surrounding communities. Some of CHCH current workers are still from the first group of twelve who took this training. They learned about the signs and symptoms of sexual abuse, and for many of them, this training opened up secrets of violence they had hidden from even their own awareness. Supported by the Resource Group, these people began to take many initiatives to spark healing in the community.

A lot of sexual abuse would happen at drinking parties, so when those working at healing heard of such a party going on, they would start to **march in the streets of the community and carry signs** saying, 'No more abuse.' They wanted to state publicly that this kind of abuse was happening and was unacceptable.

To try to break through the silence and taboos against talking about sexual abuse, they got twenty-four people who were ready to share their own stories. They mapped out the community and set out in twos or threes to speak to everyone to share their story of abuse that had happened in this community. They did this over seven days. Their stories opened the floodgates. Many disclosures followed, especially among the youth. This was an exciting but very fragile time. Victims were often blamed, and some tried to commit suicide. Many of the victimizers were in power positions in the community. The Resource Team had to figure out what to do with disclosures, how to confront victimizers, how to relate to the Western systems of justice and social services, and how to keep the community in the driver's seat of a holistic community healing movement.

The Resource Team recognized the justice system was failing them on many fronts. When victims did disclose, charges were often dropped because, when the police came to investigate, no one would talk to them due to a lack of trust. When victimizers were sent to prison, they often came back more violent and less responsible. When the victims, often children, did go to court, the justice system seemed to re-victimize them. The Resource Team saw it as their job to protect the victims and the community, especially the children, from the justice system. So, they made a new partnership with the justice system based on the needs of the community. One of the leaders of this new model called the partnership at this initial stage, the 'combination of the law and the will of the community.'

> Inherent in the Hollow Water model is the combined power of the law and the will of the community confronting abusers with the hard choice of following a healing path or facing serious consequences... (Bushie 1999, p. 12).

This partnership, named the Community Holistic Circle Healing or CHCH, developed a **13-step Healing Process** to confront abuse within the community and a protocol with the various arms of the justice and social service systems for how this would happen.

13-Step Healing Process

In each case, the team as a whole works through the 13-step process. They believe this helps to work at wholeness and to resist the fragmented and compartmentalized approach so prevalent in Western methods.

1. Disclosing - The CHCH process receives disclosures and, unlike most restorative justice initiatives, the workers investigate and work with offenders, even as they deny responsibility. At the disclosure stage, the goal is to start to attend to the needs of the victim. In two cases, the victimizer disclosed abuses they committed without a victim coming forward. If the victim is a child, the police are informed immediately. An intervention team consisting of representatives from the justice system, the child protection service, the community mental health service, and the community conducts an initial investigation. They try to determine what took place. Generally, CHCH workers do their own police work as they have developed a better trust relationship with the community than the police have. They use their own relationships with, and knowledge of, the people involved to aid in the healing process.

2. Establishing Safety for the Victim – This is done by caringly recording their story. Generally, victim's stories are believed. If the victim is a child and the victimizer is a direct family member, the child is usually taken out of the home and placed in another home within the community. This home would be a home in which the family has been trained in issues of victimization and healing. The CHCH team tries to work toward healing at every step of the process. Providing support for a victim is critical to creating the conditions to break the patterns of unhealthy relationships and to develop or strengthen healthy ones. Victims always get a worker assigned whether or not they want to work at things. This is done so the victims know they still have someone they can call.

3. Confronting the Victimizer – The first step is for the whole CHCH team to meet and plan the intervention and the confrontation of the offender. Confronting can be a long process, and the victimizer is expected to deny the offense and to use what power he or she has to control or manipulate the situation. Often, people who have previously been victimizers have the greatest potential to confront victimizers and call them to account on their denial issues. Even when victimizers admit guilt, they are not fully believed, since, in the beginning, they often only admit to small parts to avoid jail. Ultimately, the CHCH team want to make sure victimizers are serious about doing the hard work of the healing journey. The initial confrontation may take place in the person's house, a community place, a church, or sometimes out on the land where you can 'let nature do its work.' Again, the goal is to make victimizers feel safe enough to acknowledge their responsibility. The initial confrontation can take several minutes or several hours. The goal is to get the victimizers to recognize their problems. They are encouraged to admit the charges as this initiates the healing journey. Pleading guilty means that children do not need to take the stand if a case were to go to court and protects the victim from the harm of having to testify. Victimizers are given four days to decide whether to go with CHCH down the healing path or to go through the Western court system. When someone confesses, they are taken to the Royal Canadian Mounted Police (RCMP) to give a full voluntary statement about the incident and about any other abusive behavior. The RCMP charge the person just on the initially disclosed abuse and then, after having been seen by the magistrate, the person is released back to CHCH custody.

4. Supporting the Victimizers' Spouse or Parent – When the victimizer is confronted, the CHCH team fans out to those most connected to the harm. Their goal is to give everyone the same information, to begin to break the patterns of silence and manipulation, and to offer as much support as possible to those involved. The spouse naturally finds such disclosures very difficult. Some participate, consciously or not, in supporting systems of denial. Some need the care of the community as they learn such disturbing information about their spouse.

5. Supporting the Family and Community – The goal of healing is to strengthen the family and the community. The families of the victim and the victimizer are often dealing with multiple layers of harm, involving both more victims and more victimizers. Hence, dealing with abuse can trigger all kinds of other trauma. The team makes sure each family member has someone they can call after the circle closes. This is key for the healing process. Confronting the victimizers is only the beginning of the process of getting the families to shift from a blame response to a healing response that is guided by the Seven Sacred Teachings.

6. Meeting of the Assessment Team with the Police (RCMP) – The CHCH team has negotiated an arrangement with the justice system that charges are laid, but the community is given time to confront victimizers. CHCH wants to encourage victimizers to take a healing path and to demonstrate they are serious. This process can take anywhere from several months to a couple of years. Victimizers can choose to go through the court process and face jail. If they make this choice, CHCH still tries to support them and the victim. Alternatively, they can commit themselves to work on a process towards healing with CHCH, an option that does not include prison. When a victimizer commits to the healing process, the CHCH asks the courts for at least four months to determine that the victimizer is serious about healing and not just wanting to avoid jail.

7. Conducting Circles with the Victimizer – Victimizers are expected to tell their stories and work at dealing with their problems with multiple groups of people. They are also seen as out-of-balance and in need of educating about what it means to be Anishinabe, to live in balance, and to live a life guided by the Seven Sacred Teachings. The staff worker who does the initial confrontation becomes the victimizer's worker if he or she decides to work on a healing path. The first circle focuses on confession to the CHCH workers and on taking responsibility. The second circle is with the whole nuclear family and focuses on taking responsibility in this wider group. Sometimes, the second circle with the family is used to help a person move to full responsibility. The power of the relationships within the family may be enough to pull a victimizer out of denial into full responsibility. The third and final circle consists of the whole extended family. It is used to encourage the victimizer to admit guilt if he or she has not already done so and to listen to the broader community. Each circle is a time to remind people of the Seven Sacred Teachings, which underline much of the healing work. In this way, they encourage healing by rooting people in the sense of who they are as a people. A treatment plan and Healing Contract is drawn up for the victimizer. CHCH workers report that, in the last ten years, they have been using more and more traditional ceremonies as part of the plan.

8. Conducting Circles with Victim and Victimizer - By the time the victim and victimizer meet in a circle, they and their families have been working at their own speed through a long process. When the time is right, they come into a circle together. Initially, this is not a time for the victimizer to speak but for the victim to talk to the victimizer and to say what was done to them and how it has affected them. The victim's pace guides the circle. The circles are usually small, comprising two workers, the victim, and the victimizer. The CHCH team is there to 'support them, pray for them, and use the medicines.' A treatment plan is also drawn up for victims to aid in their path of healing.

9. Preparing the Families of the Victim and the Victimizer for the Sentencing Circle – Beginning four days before a Sentencing Circle happens, each night, there is a sweat ceremony in the sweat lodge. The victim and family are invited and told that the victimizer and family are also invited. If, for religious reasons, someone does not want to participate in the sweat, they are invited to come and sit outside the sweat lodge as others sweat for them. Traditionally, sweats were used for cleansing of the body, the mind, the emotions, and the Spirit; people came to bring complex conflicts and to connect with Creator.

10. Preparing the Victimizer's Family for the Sentencing Circle - The victimizer's family also is invited to participate in the sweats in preparation for the special gathering. The victimizer has many roles in preparing the sweat lodge building and in participating in traditional activities, such as 'smudging' the building to make it for healing activity. Smudging uses the smoke of sacred herbs for spiritual and emotional cleansing before Creator and is often performed before a significant gathering.

11. Conducting a Sentencing Circle – Initially, sentencing happened in the Western court, but since 1993, the community has not held its own Sentencing Circle. Here, sentencing occurs by court judge but through dialogue with the community. On the day of the event, there is a sunrise pipe ceremony, flags are hung, and the building is smudged. This is done to ask Creator to come and help. As one worker said to me:

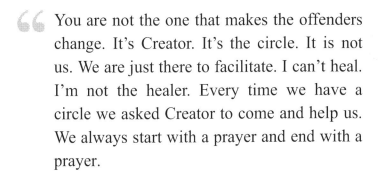 You are not the one that makes the offenders change. It's Creator. It's the circle. It is not us. We are just there to facilitate. I can't heal. I'm not the healer. Every time we have a circle we asked Creator to come and help us. We always start with a prayer and end with a prayer.

Everyone gathers in a circle. **An eagle feather** has high spiritual significance. In special gatherings, only the person who holds it has permission to speak. The eagle feather goes clockwise around the circle the first time, and everyone introduces themselves and says why they are there. The second time around, those that want to will speak to the victim in an attempt to absolve them of guilt, to build them up, and to celebrate their courage. They may also wish to transform the views of the community, which sometimes blames the victim. In the third circle of the eagle feather, the focus is on the victimizer. People are invited to share how the offence made them feel and what expectation they have of the victimizer to put things right for the victim. The fourth circle is for giving recommendations as to what needs to happen with all the people involved, for the victimizer, for the victim, and for the community. The team gives recommendations to the judge based on the whole process, but the whole community also is invited to give recommendations. In three Sentencing Circles that have occurred so far, the first of which involved 200 members of the community and the second and third involving about a 100 people each time, only one person recommended jail. The first Sentencing Circle prompted other victimizers to confess spontaneously and publicly to the community what they had done and to start a healing path. The purpose of this form of gathering is to encourage community healing and to allow the court to hear from those most affected by the victimization. The sentence comes in the form of a Healing Contract to be completed under the supervision of CHCH. Elements of that contract are spelled out in detail. Working at a Healing Contract is usually a 3 to 5-year process, which includes counseling, support groups, and multiple community circles where victimizers have to take responsibility for their efforts to date, try to understand the causes of their behavior and how their behavior affects others, and try to work toward healing with victims, extended family, and the broader community. Often, traditional ceremonies are included as part of the Healing Contract. Hollow Water's Sentencing Circle differs from some others in that it is not an attempt at community involvement at the end of a foreign process of establishing guilt. Hollow Water's Sentencing Circle is one step in a long journey of healing for the whole community. This journey started long before the Sentencing Circle, and it will have to continue long after. Here, the community marks a significant step in a healing journey for victims, for victimizers, and for the community or, alternatively, to mark the failure to try to walk a healing path. These gatherings end with everyone, including victim, victimizer and judge taking part in a feast.

12. Sentencing Review – Every six months for the duration of the Healing Contract, there is a review circle. These were started after workers realized that, after sentencing, victimizers tended to backslide, and workers did not have the resources to keep them on track. In the Sentencing Review, the community circle is reconvened, and victimizers have to answer to the broader community for their actions, rather than to the worker. The workers find this is helpful in keeping people on track.

13. Cleansing Ceremony – Before this ceremony and feast can be held, the circle of the community is reconvened to update the community on progress, to check if there are any outstanding issues or reasons they should not see this process as closed, and to work at issues of reintegration and of strengthening the community. Ceremonies mark the successful conclusion of the Healing Contract.

Over the five years of this phase, Hollow Water worked

at youth issues, alcohol abuse, sexual abuse and designed a healing program in their community that worked in partnership (including funding) with various arms of the provincial and federal government. More importantly, they started to heal from the inside.

They developed a process that recognizes the victimizer as a member of the community (rather than some Western methods that suspend the victimizer's rights as a member of the community).

As one CHCH worker put it, "You just can't give up on people. Speaking of a victimizer," she said. "He's always going to be here. His kids are here. Don't give up on this person. Keep at him or her until they understand that our focus is to one day have a healthy community."

Upon reflection on this phase, it seems to me that Hollow Water developed this process after stumbling on some critical healing insights:

- **Communities need to deal with their own harms**, rather than having them diverted to foreign systems.
- **Healing starts with the self.** Those wishing to support holistic community healing must be on a healing journey. CHCH workers are included. They have to stay sober, have to share their own stories of abuse, and need the circles of support as much as the victims and the victimizers.
- **Healing is a communal journey.**

Individualistic methods of health and justice never made sense or bore much fruit in Hollow Water. As one CHCH worker told me:

> When you go to the therapist, you walk out alone. At CHCH you don't walk out alone. We all go with you. We are all healing. When one is hurt, it affects all. Like a family.

- **Healing must shift from symptoms to root causes.** The Resource Team began by focusing on multiple symptoms having to do with youth issues and alcohol abuse. To respond meaningfully to those symptoms, they had to dig into the deeper root causes. These had to do with sexual abuse, often in childhood, and with a community journey disrupted by colonialism. Holistic community healing must create the space for victims and victimizers to work at healing their own childhood harms and, at the same time, create safe conditions for children.
- Healing Justice must be seen through **the lens of seven generations of change**. At Hollow Water, people are not only concerned with individuals. They are trying to bring an end to generations of harm by initiating generations of health and healing. Following their Anishinabe teaching, they work with longer spans of time. Seven generations is the standard measure. The teaching of Seven Generations is to understand

an action that we contemplate today by its impact on the children seven generations to come. Also, the harms of today should be understood in light of the decisions made in the past seven generations. This broader perspective does not just include the patterns and behaviors of individuals but also of communities, nations, and structures, and even of creation itself.

- '**Healing is a life-long journey, not a therapy but a way of life**.' These are the words of a CHCH worker that capture themes that came up from most people who spoke to me. Healing justice is not like retributive justice, which is supposed to be completed after you've 'done your time.' Walking a healing journey is a lifetime path and involves all areas of your life.

Phase 4: Returning To The Teachings (1994-1999)

This is the phase outsiders often refer to when speaking of Hollow Water, partly because several key reports come out of this period or reflect on it. Rupert Ross's *Return to the Teachings* and the National Film Board's film *Hollow Water* introduced the story of Hollow Water to many groups around the world. Furthermore, there were government-commissioned reports by Theresa Lajeunesse and by Couture that reported on the successes of Hollow Water reflecting on this period. Couture reported a 2% recidivism rate of those who had participated in the CHCH processes. Four Directions, an

Aboriginal justice NGO, came out with a report, which included a detailed review of the community. While there were a few criticisms offered, most notably by Lajeunesse, these reports were generally very positive. In fact, they stated there were many signs that the community was flourishing, observing the following:

- Vision for life had increased.
- Drunkenness was disappearing; the majority of the community was sober.
- Overall violence had decreased.
- Education was being completed by more people, and more were getting higher education.
- Unemployment was no longer a significant issue.
- Networking relationships outside the community had increased.
- Holistic health of children had improved.
- Community resources were broadening.
- Ownership of issues had increased.
- Ceremonies had more participants.
- Traditional ways were growing in strength.
- 'Dependency mentality' was beginning to dissipate.
- Victims reported being satisfied that they had a stake in outcomes, were feeling understood, and were fostering within themselves community and cultural pride.
- Taboos had lifted against talk about sexual abuse and dealing with it.

- Parents taught respect for others in both the nuclear and extended family contexts.
- Relocating back home to Hollow Water by band members was happening.
- Everyone now acknowledged safeness of the community.

As the community began to heal, they began to see more clearly the path they needed to follow. First, CHCH articulated a position paper on incarceration in which they listed the reasons they rejected imprisonment. These included:

- **Judgment belongs to Creator**; when used by humans it works against the healing process.
- **Incarceration does not deter offenders and does not make the community safer.**
- **Incarceration keeps people from taking responsibility**, reinforces the silence and therefore promotes, rather than breaks, the cycle of violence.
- **A legal system with a lengthy process which presumes innocence until guilt is proven means no accountability, and it sets the conditions for re-offending**.
- **People return from jail having been put out of balance** by being told that 'they have paid for their crime;' now, out of balance and believing that they are done, they are more dangerous to the community than before they went in.

Second, and intimately related to the first, CHCH saw that holistic community healing required them to return to the traditional teachings. This return to tradition has been a slow movement because the community had been so thoroughly traumatized that the traditional teachings have been forgotten, or at least those who remembered did not feel safe in sharing them. Some of the churches in Hollow Water have taught that traditional things are evil, while others have encouraged and participated in traditional ceremonies. In the beginning, Elders from other communities had to be brought in to help them remember their traditions and create the space where they might practice these traditions. Even now, for many of the victims and victimizers, the first time they hear of the traditional teachings is when they get involved with the CHCH program. In trying to return to a more traditional path, the people at Hollow Water turned wherever they could to find help. Sometimes, this was the Cree - at times a historic enemy-, sometimes, people from across the US border and, sometimes, from other Anishinabe. They pieced together a traditional approach that fits their identity and is similar to the Anishinabe of pre-colonial times. Today, many CHCH workers report going to both church and traditional ceremonies. For some, this had been a difficult balance in the past but has become more acceptable.

The 13-step process did not change much during this phase, but the supporting ethos became more rooted in traditional ways. Members of the healing movement brought back the sweat lodge, pipe ceremonies, and smudging. Just walking through the offices and surrounding grounds, I noticed many signs of traditional practices. A large teepee was set up outside the offices. Behind it was a sweat lodge. Out towards the woods was the traditional ceremony ground with flags on trees, community fire circles and, inside the woods, traditional fasting and vision quest grounds. For many CHCH workers, traditional culture is the source of life and the source of the healing journey. The ceremonies represent the teachings woven into the physical surroundings. As one Elder put it:

> To us, ceremonies and everyday life can never be separated. It is a complete package. It's not religion. It can't be separated.

The Sweat Lodge is used for cleansing the person and the community. One worker explained to me that the sweat lodge helps them spiritually by giving them the strength to continue the healing path. They do not seem to expect a shortcut on the healing path, to be healed instantly and entirely. But they do expect the traditional culture to be a source of much healing.

In Hollow Water, CHCH workers also work with Christian community members who are not interested in traditional culture. They find ways of supporting their Christian spiritual journey, so the physical, emotional, spiritual, and mental are all in balance, thus applying a traditional insight in 'non-traditional' ways.

Other traditional activities include **The Sacred Fir**e, which is a quarterly community activity that begins and ends with a community feast. This fire is kept alive for four days for prayers for healing. Once a year, the community also celebrates **Black Island Days**. Black Island is an island nearby where most of the community goes for a week of the summer. Here, they sleep in tents and organize various activities. Alcohol is not allowed. Community members report that 'everything is different there' and that 'people just automatically care for each other's kids, there are kids that come with no food and others just take care of them.' Black Island Days is a time of being together on their traditional grounds, a community close to creation.

Victims, victimizers, and the whole community were encouraged to participate in these activities as part of their healing. Healing includes learning who you are and how you are connected to the rest of the world. For the workers and for those they were working with, this traditional approach bore much fruit. Sentencing Circles in 1993, 1995, and 1998 were large community events and included a number of traditional elements that were offered as options to participants.

Although some see CHCH as an alternative justice program, the workers of CHCH now see their work as returning the community to traditional ways. This return includes doing justice in ways that come out of their traditions. However, it is a problem when victimizers see CHCH as an alternative to the incarceration program. They want victimizers to get to the point where they are serious about healing, not just avoiding incarceration. They want victims and victimizers to get to a point where they can be a healing resource to the broader community, rather than seeing the abuse as something dealt with by a program of experts. CHCH works because it is rooted in a holistic, spiritual vision.

Community holistic healing became more about returning to the traditions and learning to live in the way of the ancestors, that is, with love, respect, and a strong sense of identity as Anishinabe. In Hollow Water, healing is not a program or project that could be done by a small set of experts. Healing is the work of Creator. It is a spiritual practice where community members can facilitate the coming together of the circle, but it is clear that Creator is the source of healing justice.

During this phase, healing justice was well-researched and reported to be more effective than anything else in Canada in working with sexual abuse victims. All the studies during this phase showed evidence of some measure of success.

Phase 5: Momentum Sliding (1999-2006)

Over this eight-year period, the healing movement at Hollow Water went into a backward slide, even as it continued to broaden its approach to healing.

There were two key indicators of this slide. First was that **Sentencing Circles** stopped. When I was there, the last one was in 1998, and they were trying to plan one for 2007. Second, sexual abuse disclosures stopped. From 2002-2006, there were no sexual abuse disclosures, signifying the community no longer felt safe or trusted the CHCH workers. These are devastating marks of problems for a holistic community healing movement, meaning the community's partial withdrawal of participation in the movement.

I asked many questions to try to understand this slide and heard many different ideas.

Concerning Sentencing Circles, there were victimizers ready and waiting for circles to happen. But Sentencing Circles didn't occur. As the circles were crucial times of healing, this seemed to facilitate the community slide. Part of the reason for the lack of circles seems to be a breakdown in the relationship with the Western justice system. Funding from the justice system has continued but is still at 1993 levels as of Fall 2006. Moreover, significant figures in the system that worked with the community in earlier phases are no longer there, and

CHCH workers feel there is less understanding with new officials.

CHCH also went through a significant leadership transition in 1999 when one of the founding leaders left the program, but not the community, for another job. The new leader had a different style and perhaps different priorities. CHCH started to be restructured more hierarchically. The CHCH morale, which had been quite high, began to slip. Bickering and gossip increased. Use of circles for workers to support each other decreased. New people were hired but without clear roles, orientation, training, or mentoring. Some workers got into an 'I'm not paid to do that' mind-set. Initially, wages had been the same for everyone, but that started to change as some workers completed Bachelor of Social Work programs in 2000. The disparities created friction with other workers. Some workers went into reproduction mode, trying to reproduce their previous successes without learning new things and inviting people to come and be involved in the growing movement. Some workers no longer seemed to follow a healing journey personally, and the boundaries of acceptable behavior for a CHCH worker were pushed as at least one worker admitted to using drugs and alcohol when off work.

CHCH was a program within Child and Family Services (CFS) and was housed in the same building. In 2005, the director of CFS felt the pressure for change from staff, so CFS was relocated from CHCH offices to the Band and Council offices. This was a highly visible marker that those who talked about healing and health could not get along. When Burma Bushie was rehired as Coordinator of CHCH, her role was different from her previous time in leadership. The Resource Team, a cross-section of the community supporting the work, was gone. So were other leaders who had shared particular areas of responsibility. Some looked to Burma to be the single spearhead to re-engage the community movement. But a single leader could not dictate holistic community healing. Besides, Burma was ill. Reeling from its split, the program continued to struggle. In a 2006 envisioning workshop I attended, CHCH admitted the poor relationship with CFS and Band Council was fuelling mistrust and confusion in the community. CHCH had lost much integrity and credibility.

Continued Marks of Healing and Growth

However, during this time, CHCH continued to expand its ways of doing healing. In 2001, they recovered the traditional summer ceremony that includes a four-day vision quest and fasts from all food and water. Those who choose to can fast for their health or the health of the community. These fasts and vision quests have been held each of the last six years. People report the fast helps to heal by creating a time to connect with Creator and to reflect on the interconnections within creation. A number reported having visions, mostly of people who had died and, perhaps, whom they needed to let go, to forgive, or to receive encouragement. It is a time to slow down and connect with spiritual things.

CHCH introduced four new programs during this time:

- **Wilderness Therapy** - This program takes mostly youth and young adults into the wilderness as part of educating people of healthier ways of living and reconnecting them with traditional activities. They camp together, hunt, listen to Elders, and sometimes work with the dog sled teams as a way of healing. In these settings, people reconnect with the land, the Elders, and ultimately with Creator. Some trips are organized with the school while others are more informal in organization. Some links are made between victimizers and victims, who are both encouraged to be part of the wilderness program and the dog teams. CHCH workers and school staff testify that these times in the wilderness have a profound healing effect.
- **Sewing Club** - Sewing Club is an informal time for Elders to get together. The process of doing traditional activities also encourages them to talk about things that happened to them.
- **Traditional Dance** - This program, started in 2005, reintroduces Powwow dancing and singing into the community. This dancing is for exercise, but CHCH sees it as helping people find their traditional identity through practicing

dance as a sacred bond between a dancer and Creator. Some of those who have been initiated into the Powwow circle have gone on to learn their traditional names, get their colors, and learn their clan, all marks of Anishinabe identity. The hope is that such rootedness in identity leads to respectful living.

- **Returning to Spirit Trainings (RTS)** - RTS is a training that Hollow Water has borrowed. It is a resource set up to help Aboriginal communities heal from the abuse and fall out of Residential Schools. Many CHCH workers are taking this training and point towards it as one of the sources of hope and motivation for their work. Through a series of five-day training, RTS looks at issues of disempowerment and life patterns based in brokenness and builds toward concrete ways of letting go and building a positive identity.

CHCH works in partnership with the local school on some projects, such as health week, quarterly health symposiums, wilderness therapy programs, and art therapy. It also encourages the school's Anishinabe language-immersion program.

Expanding Vision of Holistic Healing

As the practices of healing justice have grown, so has the vision. While their vision has always been a holistic community vision, as members of Hollow Water have matured in their healing and deepened their rootedness in traditional ways, they have come to articulate the healing journey to be one of nation-building and self-sufficiency. Sometimes, this is communicated as economic or community development, but these concepts are used to point back towards a particular kind of nationhood. They recognize the community is hugely dependent on the government. The dependency is created through the welfare system, which they estimate includes 60% of the community, but also through the Indian Act, which mandates particular kinds of governance, and through CHCH, which is funded by the government. They desire to create an economic base where they do not have to rely on the government. They recognize it is insufficient to try to help people heal from the pain of abuse and colonialization and to advocate healthy ways of living when people cannot get a job.

Note that, for the Hollow Water healing movement, nationhood is quite distinct from the nation-state. They are not seeking equality of power with the Western state system. For at least some of them, both the state system and the notion of equality are based on a conception of violent power. As explained to me, equality seeks to find a balance between two negatives: too much power and not enough. Both too much and too little power result in violence. As one Elder put it:

66 What I am talking about is based on a right

spirit and the intent of creation. It doesn't give anyone special rights – it is that power piece that has no place in what I am talking about. It is a birthright, a birth responsibility. Until that is back in place, we will always be struggling. That is one of the things that we have to put right.

For the Anishinabe of Hollow Water, healing seems to be about rediscovering their birthright and birth responsibility as part of Creator's good creation.

This phase from 1999-2006 is one of backsliding and building at the same time. The healing movement seems almost critically wounded while, at the same time, learning to soar. Basic elements in the healing journey were side-lined, and the impact was profound and immediate. When the healing path is not regularly tended, it starts to slip.

Phase 6: Searching For The Healing Path Again (2006-Continuing)

Backsliding, brokenness, and darkness might constitute a critical blow for other communities, but not so in Hollow Water, at least not yet. Hollow Water knows darkness and brokenness all too well. While some report it feels like they are back to where they were fifteen years ago, Hollow Water has a longer record of cultivating holistic community healing. The lessons learned along the way equip them to find the path again.

When even somewhat discouraged CHCH workers are asked how far they have come in the healing journey, they identify many signs of health:

- '**Women are stronger**. They can stand up and say I don't need to have this kind of a life. I don't need to be beaten.'
- '**More than half of the community has been involved in CHCH**, but maybe even the whole community, as we are all related here.'
- 'We are a small community surrounded by the Métis community. **These communities are coming together. This is part of the healing path.** I remember when I was growing up there was lots of open fighting between the communities.'
- '**You walk around the community, and you see traditional things now – sweat lodges – that never used to be the case**.'

I asked one Elder if there was anyone who was beyond the possibility of being restored. He paused, then he said, 'I don't know. I haven't seen it yet.' Then he gave a good laugh. Hollow Water has looked into the eyes of the darkest kinds of abuses but has not yet found someone who could not be restored. If this is true for individuals, perhaps it is true for communities.

While I visited CHCH, they had two days of re-envisioning. Four Directions International facilitated their efforts to understand where the community stood regarding the healing movement and what steps CHCH could take to build support. They articulated the following ten steps:

- Enlarge and transform the circle of CHCH management or governance.
- Re-engage the community; it is the support base.
- Continue culturally based programming.
- Conduct targeted healing campaigns (for sexual abuse, drugs, alcohol).
- Work to heal critical relationships with political leaders and CFS.
- Bring healing into the context of nation building.
- Develop a stable funding base.
- Create enterprise to pay for social development.
- Care for yourself; healing begins with the circle of workers.
- Hold the plan to account.

It is too early to be sure, but perhaps, these plans represent a new phase on the healing journey. CHCH workers seemed cautiously optimistic. After an eight-year hiatus, they and justice system workers planned a Sentencing Circle in Hollow Water.

Despite the decline described above, I was inspired by

my time with the CHCH workers and listening to their stories. They have a deep commitment to protecting children and to healing their community. Furthermore, they have touched and tasted what healing justice is like. What is unclear is where the path ahead will lead.

What sustains the Hollow Water experience of healing justice? The ups and downs of their own story is good evidence of what helps to sustain healing justice and what acts as a barrier when neglected.

Nine dynamics seem most important. They are listed in the order of frequency in which they were discussed in interviews, ranging from 100% for themes listed first to 60% for those listed last.

Returning to Creator and Traditional Culture

The source of healing justice is listening to and being in **relationship with Creator**. This does not mean that those who do not acknowledge Creator cannot experience healing. Nevertheless, a human program divorced from its roots will struggle to bear good fruit. When the Resource Group began to meet in the 1980s, they did not set out to re-establish traditional culture. However, they discovered along the way that many of the decisions they had made followed traditional understandings (e.g., healing begins with the self). In Hollow Water, healing justice is sustained through the traditional ceremonies and protocols. It is also supported through their **tradi-**

tional language. One Elder explained it to me in these terms:

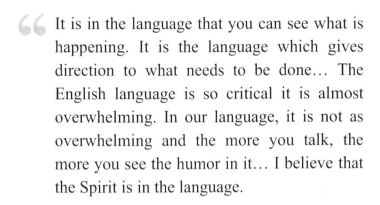 It is in the language that you can see what is happening. It is the language which gives direction to what needs to be done... The English language is so critical it is almost overwhelming. In our language, it is not as overwhelming and the more you talk, the more you see the humor in it... I believe that the Spirit is in the language.

Recovery of the traditional culture means restoring the role of Elders and women and recovering the traditional practices of sweats, feasts, and ceremonies. It also means recovering a sense of traditional practices of governance and food production. More and more of the CHCH workers are also wondering if the recovering of the clan system is a necessary part of moving back to stable structures. Recovery of these things does not mean going back to the way it was as if the world had not kept changing. It does mean creating the space where traditions that were interrupted and disturbed have an opportunity to speak to the dynamics of today.

Staying Close to Creation

One CHCH worker told me 'Change comes in part from being close to creation.' This theme arose in every interview. Staying close to creation is closely connected with traditional culture. To find the Good Life, to find a healing path, one must find a path that respects the vast interdependencies of creation. Healing is a way of living in balance with one's self, community, and with all creation. Anything that harms the balance of relationships in creation leads to suffering, an unbalanced life. Anything that respects those relationships leads to healing and the Good Life. As Hollow Water has matured in healing practices, they have found more ways to encourage the community to stay close to creation. Black Island Days, the Wilderness Therapy Program, the ceremonies, the fasts, the sacred fire are all of this type of healing rooted in staying close to the land.

Connecting the Community

Healing is sustained when the community comes together in a circle to explore healing together. In the early days of CHCH, they focused on sharing stories of abuse that happened in the community. Those first circles created a momentum sustained by the consistent circles of the Resource Team. The 13-step process is a process of ever-expanding circles where each circle reflects together on what it means to take responsibility, to walk a healing path, to follow the Seven Sacred Teachings, to be Anishinabe. Loss of momentum in healing followed the failure to gather: as the Resource Team, as Sentencing Circles, and as regular staff circles. When the community no longer gathers in these circles, then the healing movement slides.

Preferring the Local

The healing path only started to open up when a group recognized that the outside systems were making the community sicker and that they had to find ways to take community healing back into their hands. From time to time, they had to decide on what this would look like. CHCH had an uneasy relationship with some of the outside professionals. A psychologist, working from her training and understanding of best practices, strongly cautioned the program against bringing victim and victimizers into the same circle. CHCH workers followed her advice until some children pushed them to interact with their parents who were their victimizers. By following the local ways of knowing and sometimes breaking the Western best practice rules, Hollow Water discovered a path of healing that is unparalleled in Canada.

Staying Close to Suffering

Those involved in the healing movement shared their stories and created space for others to do the same. CHCH workers, when at their best, do not work as paid staff but as family members engaging with their community. Whereas earlier victims had been blamed and victimizers exported to the criminal justice system, CHCH created space for both to stay to share their stories, to walk a healing path, and even to become a healing resource for their community. As one long-term CHCH worker put it:

> 66 I think one of the reasons why we can reach offenders is because we treat them like family, like human beings, like you and me. They have feelings. They have pains. We don't shun them or push them away. We treat them like family and talk to them. You have to be tough with them but also to treat them like human beings.

When victims and victimizers are not treated like family, healing deteriorates. However, when a community finds creative ways to stay close to those who are suffering and treat them like family, it seems that surprising healing paths start to unfold. This dynamic even extends to the CHCH workers. When CHCH workers no longer treat each other as family, healing slides.

Special Role of Women and Children

Most CHCH workers said that what keeps them going in their work is their children and grandchildren. The women of Hollow Water see it as their traditional responsibility to protect children. As the women have stood up to protect children, they have grown stronger. As they have listened to the children, they have also been challenged and shaped to follow more radical healing paths. This second dynamic of the special role of children and women has helped to sustain the healing movement over the last twenty years.

Training and Supporting the Team

The healing path is sustained by learning together and healing together. A breakthrough happened in the healing movement as a consequence of community members committing to a two-year training course. Regular support meetings with the Resource Team also served this function and led to an ethos of CHCH workers supporting each other through circles. At various points in their history, trainings were hosted to engage people in learning about abuse and healing. When that support and accountability started to slide, so did the healing movement. CHCH workers are clear that, when at their best, they work not as experts but as people who are also on a healing journey. When they stop working at their own healing, they lose integrity and the trust of the community.

Funding Barriers

CHCH is funded by provincial funds of $120,000 per year and federal funds of $120,000 per year. Initially, this was to cover the salaries of seven sexual abuse workers and one secretary. While CHCH has grown through the years, funding levels have never increased. Funding was not even raised after a government-commissioned report on the cost-benefit analysis reported that, for every $2 spent in Hollow Water, $6-$15 in direct cost was saved. Also, there were tremendous benefits that could not be quantified in dollar amounts. The result is that CHCH worker salaries have not changed since the early 1990s, except that those who completed university degrees were given a raise. When I was there, Hollow Water had some additional funding from the Aboriginal Healing Foundation, but those funds are a term grant and not stable core funding. CHCH workers say the healing path would be better sustained by allowing for regular salary increases.

Hollow Water is also faced with a long-term challenge of what funding should look like in their community. To follow the path of self-sufficiency and nation-building might mean funding that is not dependent on Western systems. Within traditional Anishinabe teachings, spiritual matters - like healing - should not be commoditized. Working out what this means in today's world of money is one of their challenges.

Healing Creates More Healing

At Hollow Water, people took a step and did something, even when they didn't understand fully what they were doing. As one CHCH worker said, 'Going out and doing it created more healing.' Although there are times when CHCH seems to get stuck in ideas and planning, the healing path seems to flourish when they find a way to take a further step on a healing path. Healing is a resource that seems to multiply when used, like yeast.

When the community (and workers) taste it, they find the courage to take more steps.

Barriers To Healing Justice In Hollow Water

Hollow Water's healing movement has faced many obstacles along the way. Besides neglect of the dynamics listed above, there have been other impediments. When asked about these, respondents spoke of both external and internal barriers. The process of colonialization set up external obstacles that still impact the community.

Electing Chief and Council

An electoral system was imposed on Aboriginal communities in Canada through the Indian Act. The traditional methods of recognizing leadership within the community were displaced by order of electing leaders, which were more familiar by Western standards. This system was imposed as part of the policy of assimilation or what Couture calls cultural genocide. In other words, the current electoral system in Hollow Water was not designed on healing principles. It is not surprising this system then mitigates healing in the community. CHCH relationship with Chief and Council has been better or worse, depending on who is in power, but the point about this barrier is not just about who is there. Elections every two years leaves the community divided. Furthermore, those community members who rise to the top of such leadership structures often are those that use hierarchical power, further complicating efforts to make healing a community-wide initiative. Notably, while women are the substantial majority of CHCH workers, they are very much a minority among elected leaders.

Weakening Relationships with Western Justice System

Although part of what makes the Hollow Water program innovative is its partnership with the Western justice system, this partnership has been strained at many points. Those in Hollow Water feel neither supported nor understood by the justice system. The low funding rates and the inability to organize a Sentencing Circle for eight years are evidence of this stain and this barrier for healing. It seems that CHCH either needs a more supportive relationship with the justice system or a more independent one. It is not clear which road they will take or whether these roads are mutually exclusive.

Welfare System That Supports Poverty

The welfare system supports many people in Hollow Water and, some would say, they are dependent on it. CHCH workers realize it is easier to stay on welfare than to go to work. But they believe this dependency affects a person's sense of identity in negative ways, which can make them more prone towards abuse and less inclined towards healing. Healing is about learning to value your identity. When that personal identity is devalued by a dependency system, like the welfare system, the healing path becomes more difficult.

Church Relationships

The relationship of the healing movement with churches has also gone up and down, depending on the church denomination and who is in leadership. From the beginning, there have been churches that teach traditional ways are evil, thus creating a barrier for some to work with CHCH. There are also churches that have supported CHCH from the beginning and have participated in the Resource Group and in ceremonies.

Incarceration

"The Hollow Water Position on Incarceration" paper names incarceration as a barrier to healing. Of course, confinement was not designed to promote healing. The Anishinabe perspective is that healing must be the basis for their community structures, as well as the healing process. Incarceration interrupts this process. It takes people out of the community and returns them, sometimes, more dangerous than when they left. Furthermore, the language around incarceration is that once you have 'done your time, you've paid your debt.' This language runs counter to the need for healing, for taking responsibility, for making things right to the victim, for learning about identity, and for offering your gifts to the community.

In addition to the external barriers mentioned above, there are some internal barriers.

Keeping the Secret

When CHCH started, one of the most significant impediments was the internal dynamic of keeping secrets. Sexual abuse was a taboo subject, but the majority of community members were directly affected in some way. To work at healing on this matter was to reveal secrets that had been carefully hidden. Many people did not want to admit there was a problem. Some even tried harming the CHCH workers. While these dynamics are changing, the absence of sexual abuse disclosures since 2002 is evidence that this is a barrier the community continues to face.

Top-down and Diffuse Leadership

There have been times when leaders within CHCH imposed top-down leadership and times when others have looked to single leaders to organize the whole community on a healing path. Then the healing path has suffered. On the other hand, there is an Aboriginal culture of not wanting to tell people what to do but expecting everyone to do their work. I have called this 'diffuse leadership.' Hollow Water needs to create a new style of leadership that respects the culture and their understanding of healing. What seems clear is that strictly top-down and diffuse styles of leadership create barriers for the movement.

Relationship with Children and Family Services

CFS and CHCH were woven together from the beginning. The 2005 split of these two organizations created major barriers to the healing movement. One part of the barrier impedes the flow of information and the need to work together on cases involving children who are under the CFS mandate. Another part is the loss of trust of the community in the workers when the healing movement is threatened with messy public breakups.

Workers Are Not Walking a Healing Path

When the community perceives CHCH workers as not walking a healing path, then healing seems to slide. Sometimes, this happens by workers falling into gossip. Sometimes, it is the failure to convene circles to help and support each other. Another example is the breakdown of the relationship between CHCH and CFS. There is at least one CHCH worker who admitted to using alcohol and drugs when not working. In the past, CHCH workers were the ones who became sober. This was seen as a requirement of employment, and some people were dismissed for not following this guideline. CHCH's inability to envision an appropriate response seemed to some a mark of their weakness. That issue may have gone away, as the last reports at the time of writing were that the worker was addressing personal health issues and no longer using drugs. However, the broader question of how to support and encourage CHCH workers to stay on a healing path is an issue that will not go away.

Guilt and Shame

Hollow Water has identified guilt and shame as 'emotional blocks, so the person doesn't grow.' Both lead to paralysis, not healing. Consequently, at each step in the

CHCH process, the workers try to remove guilt and shame. The whole community needs to learn that the victims are not to blame but need a release from guilt and shame. Furthermore, they need healing and maybe the offer of a healing path and a support worker. The same understandings apply to the victimizers.

Being Labelled a Process or Project

CHCH recognizes that one of the most significant obstacles to holistic healing is seeing and treating CHCH as a process or project. CHCH is an alliance of a broad section of the community. It is not narrowly focused as an alternative justice program but is about holistic community healing. Partly because the program has paid workers, some see it as a model where a few experts are responsible, not the community. However, taking the community off the hook is a massive barrier to sustaining a community holistic healing movement. When the community has not taken responsibility, the healing movement has started to slide.

Losing Creator

66 What happens when we stop acknowledging Creator? We suffer. We go through that darkness in our community. That's the battle in this community; it is when we forget Creator. It's like going off that path and into a mess. That is when the red flag goes up. That is when a person can do all these crimes.

> Because he is not connected to Creator and not connected to any kinship, family breakdown starts to happen.

I learned from Elders that people are seen as the instruments, but **it is Creator who does the healing**. However, there seems to be a tendency to forget Creator, to forget to give thanks for the good things, and to do only your own work. The Elders said, when this happens, all sorts of trouble follows.

Final Words

The story of Hollow Water is one of the strongest stories of healing justice in the Canadian context. However, it is also a story full of ups and downs.

THE FRAGILITY in their story suggests to me that healing justice is not a robust process to be adopted but is more like a fragile plant to be carefully tended.

THEIR UPS and downs can teach us a lot about what is needed to sustain healing justice. Their story also shines a spotlight on barriers that can hinder a holistic community healing movement.

Chapter 4 - The Iona Community and the Wild Goose

A Touching Place

To the lost Christ shows his face
to the unloved he gives his embrace
to those who cry in pain or disgrace
Christ makes, with his friends, a touching place.

Christ's is the world in which we move
Christ's are the folk we're summoned to love
Christ's is the voice that calls us to care
and Christ is the one who meets us there.

Feel for the people we most avoid
strange or bereaved or never employed
feel for the women and feel for the men
who fear that their living is all in vain.

Feel for the parents who've lost their child
feel for the women whom men have defiled
feel for the baby for whom there's no breast
and feel for the weary who find no rest.

Feel for the lives by life confused
riddled with doubt, in loving abused
feel for the lonely heart, conscious of sin
which longs to be pure but fears to begin
(Bell and Maule 1986).

Not many songs of worship in the Christian lexicon focus on social misfits, the unemployed, rape victims, motherless children, and others crying in pain. Somehow, the dysfunctions and excesses of social, economic, and political structures do not seem to have a significant place in much Christian worship and, perhaps, theology. One of the exceptions to this tendency is the music coming out of the Iona Community's **Wild Goose Resource Group**, such as the song quoted above, which was written by John Bell, a member of the Iona Community, and Graham Maule, a former member and staff person.

These songs of worship are rare and come out of a particular orientation to God, to the world and, indeed, to justice. This particular kind of justice finds its place in the intermingling of healing, politics, spirituality, work, geography, prayer, non-violent action, ecological peace-building, and worship. Kathy Galloway, a former leader of the community, has called this kind of justice, a 'justice that heals.'

The Iona Community, founded in Scotland in 1938, is a dispersed network of Christian peace and justice activists. Mostly urban, this community has survived two critical transitions: the transition from a very charismatic founding leader and the transition required when there were no longer any of the founding members among them. When I spent time with them, the Iona Community had about 250 members, dispersed mostly in Britain, and over 1500 Associates and 1400 friends.

But what do they mean by a justice that heals? What are practices of healing justice present in this mostly white, urban, and dispersed Christian community? What have they learned about what sustains and blocks such a justice?

Because the Iona Community is a community that values diversity, a wide range of views and practices exists within its membership. Their views sometimes conflict. I have tried to capture themes from multiple sources within the Community in the hope that such ideas are broadly reflective of the group. However, you should understand that 'the Iona Community' does not refer to a uniform community but a diverse one.

To understand how the Iona Community approaches healing justice, it is necessary to understand their history. In 1938, the Rev. George MacLeod, founder and first Leader of the Iona Community, set off to the **Scottish**

Isle of Iona on an experiment. MacLeod, a soldier turned pacifist minister in an inner-city congregation of the Church of Scotland in Glasgow, was convinced the church was mostly irrelevant to the life and struggles of the industrialized inner city, a place so often marked by poverty and by the structural failings of the industrialized world. He was also convinced that the way the world tried to solve problems through violent means, in fact, explained few of the underlying issues. As one member told me, MacLeod was touched by double-edged injustice: the injustice of poverty, which made people feel worthless and ashamed, and the injustice of a church that had lost touch with the poor and lost its true vocation. This criticism of the structural injustice of church and world has continued in the Iona Community. MacLeod believed the world needed alternative ways of doing politics and economics and of dealing with conflict. The Iona Community was developed to help build this alternative politics. The first focus was on transforming those who were leading the church. The way to change the church was to change the way it trained ministers. So, when MacLeod went to the Scottish Isle of Iona, he took with him a few ministers-in-training and a few unemployed craftsmen. Their task was to rebuild the Abbey buildings while living together in Christian community. Here lay the beginnings of the Iona Community.

In some ways, **the Abbey on the Isle of Iona** is a symbol of the life of the Iona Community. To understand the Community, it is necessary to know something of the historical and theological shoulders on which they stand. The Abbey was originally built in 1208, when Reginald, Lord of Isles, invited the Benedictine order to establish a community on Iona. This order of the Western Church emphasized the role of prayer, community worship, work, scholarship, hospitality, and the unity of the church. However, the Benedictines were not the first to establish a Christian community on Iona. The foundations of the Abbey lie on the ruins of St. Columba's monastery. Columba came from Ireland to Iona in 563 and established a community of monks that, in its **Celtic tradition**, emphasized hospitality, healing, love for all creation and regular corporate worship. In those early years, Iona was a center of Celtic spirituality. Today, Celtic spirituality plays a vital role in the Iona Community. While it does not see itself strictly as a Celtic community, it does present itself as a community with 'Scottish roots and international membership.' The publishing house of the community is called **Wild Goose Publications. The wild goose is the Celtic symbol for the Holy Spirit.** J. Philip Newell, former Warden at the Abbey and an Associate of the Iona Community, contrasts the key characteristics of Celtic spirituality with the Mediterranean church based in Rome.

> Two major features of the Celtic tradition distinguish it from what in contrast can be called the 'Mediterranean' tradition. Celtic spirituality is marked by the belief that **what is deepest in us is the image of God.** Sin has

distorted and obscured that image but not erased it. The Mediterranean tradition, on the other hand, in its doctrine of original sin has taught that what is deepest in us is our sinfulness. This has given rise to a tendency to define ourselves regarding the ugliness of our sin instead of the beauty of our origins. **The second major characteristic of the Celtic tradition is a belief in the essential goodness of creation.** Not only is creation viewed as a blessing, but it is also regarded as a theophany or a showing of God. Thus the great Celtic teachers refer to it as 'the book of creation' in which we may read the mystery of God. The Mediterranean tradition, on the other hand, has tended towards a separation of spirit and matter and thus has distanced the mystery of God from the matter of creation.

This view of Christianity is reflected in some fascinating ways in the Iona Community.

However, the spiritual history of Iona is not exclusive to the Celts and the Benedictines. Before the Celts, the site was sacred to the Druids. After the Celts and Benedictines had come and gone, the island, including the Abbey precincts, came into the ownership of the Duke of Argyll. In 1899, the ruins of the abbey were placed by him into the hands of the Church of Scotland Trustees with the agreement that the Abbey church be restored, and all branches of the Christian Church should be able to worship there. This long history of Iona being sacred ground is also evidenced by the kinds of people who lie in the ancient graveyard: 48 Scottish kings, eight Norwegian kings, and some Irish and French monarchs.

So, the Isle of Iona and its Abbey have a long tradition of being a sacred place that emphasizes hospitality, communal worship, common work, Christian unity, and care for all creation. The history of the Abbey and of Iona has immense symbolic significance for the Iona Community.

While the island and the Abbey are symbolic of the life of the Iona Community, they are not the focus. The community has always had three key avenues of action: **the two island centers of Iona and Mull**, its **headquarters in Glasgow**, and its **members dispersed around the world** (but mostly in Britain). The 250 Members and 2900 Associates and Friends are considered the core of the Iona Community. These members are the hands and feet of the community around the world. They run their island centers as demonstration plots of life in response to God.

Since the original vision was to train ministers, the Iona Community is not organized as a congregation or primarily as a geographic community. The Iona Community is not a church. Membership was initially open only to Church of Scotland ministers-in-training and therefore only to men. Over time, the craftsmen, who were working and rebuilding the Abbey alongside the minsters-in-training, felt excluded from the organization, so membership was made open to laypeople and, later still, to women. Slowly opening the doors of the community has been part of the community's journey to healing justice. It has moved from initially excluding women to fully including women. When I was with them, The Leader of the Community was female. Initially, members were expected to spend summers at the island of Iona, working along with the craftsmen at rebuilding and living in a simple community that worshiped and studied the Bible together. After a few months on the island, they were expected to go back to the city, often to housing projects in low-income areas of Glasgow. In fact, they committed themselves to working for two years in an urban parish.

Today, members are expected to spend a week on the Island and to participate in three plenary sessions (one of which is held regionally). What holds the community together is its five-fold commitment. **The Rule** that each member commits to includes:

1. Daily prayer and Bible reading
2. Sharing and accounting for the use of money
3. Planning and accounting for the use of time
4. Acting for justice and peace in society
5. Meeting with and being accountable to each other.

The island centers are built on the small islands of Iona and Mull off the coast of Scotland. Their setting in a beautiful rugged land plays a significant role in the life of the community. Many have described Iona as 'a thin place' where only a tissue separates the material from the spiritual.

On the Isle of Iona is the Abbey, which houses the 25 or so resident staff and the over 100 volunteers who come for various periods over the summer. The Warden and as few as two members live on the island year-round. The island is significant, but it is not the main location of community. It is a place to host people and to teach them about the vision and practices of the Iona Community. The Abbey hosts up to 48 visitors, who come for short courses. They participate in all areas of community life, doing the dishes, eating together, sharing in worship planning or in music, crafts, drama, and social events.

The MacLeod Centre, also on Iona, was opened in 1988. This center accommodates 40 people. This island center also runs particular courses or programs. Between the two centers, they can host almost 100 people per week through the program period. In 2007, the year of my visit, they scheduled over 60 programs with themes covering a range of topics, including peacemaking, non-violence, young adults, liturgical celebrations, spirituality of land, Christian spiritual practice, pilgrimage, Black liberation theology, poverty and social justice, non-discrimination and sexuality, faith in politics, money and wealth, music festivals, God and the city, and interfaith and interdenominational dialogues.

Camas, a third program center on the Isle of Mull, is about three miles from the Isle of Iona and is a center for young people to come for adventure holidays in a Christian environment. Traditionally, youth have come from inner-city Glasgow but also from many other areas. Camas is also the setting where the community hosts young offenders in custody at Polmont Institute. They come to the center to experience a simple lifestyle in tune with the local environment. While the centers operate on a break-even basis, the Abbey shop, Wild Goose Publications, and the contributions of Members, Associates and Friends provide the bulk of the funding for the whole organization.

In Glasgow, Scotland the community has a publishing house, **Wild Goose Publications**, a **Wild Goose Resource and Worship Group**, a **Youth Department**, and the **administrative base** from which they operate a **bi-monthly magazine, *Coracle*.**

Members work in a variety of jobs, about one-third working as ministers, priests, and chaplains, and two-thirds working in other spheres of service, such as health, education, justice advocacy, and social service. Members are dispersed around the world. They participate in a wide range of churches, and some do not identify with any particular church. They are organized into family groups and regional groups that are geographically based. Family groups are the context of support and accountability in following the Rule of Iona. These groups are arranged as geographic clusters. Individual members follow the annual Iona guide for daily prayer. They also do regular Bible reading and figure out within their context how to live in the commitment for action for peace and justice in society.

During its almost seventy years, the focus of the Community has shifted and grown. When I was there, they had eight areas of focus:

- Justice, peace, and the integrity of creation (opposing nuclear weapons, campaigning against the arms trade and for **ecological justice**)
- Political and cultural action to **combat racism**
- Action for **economic justice**, locally, nationally and globally
- Issues in **human sexuality**
- Discovery of new and relevant **approaches to worship**
- Work with young people
- Deepening of **ecumenical dialogue and communion**
- **Inter-faith relations**

Many of these areas have dedicated working groups of Iona Community members. They work to develop and promote their themes within the Community through plenary meetings, beyond their own membership through hosting workshops at the island centers or by partnering with groups of like minds.

Within the international church, the Iona Community is perhaps best known for its **worship resources in the form of songs, liturgies, and dramas.** The Iona Community is a singing community and has shared the songs and worship resources they have collected and written through the Wild Goose Resource and Worship Group.

However, this reputation for worship resources is somewhat misleading. Those resources come out of visions and practices of justice, healing, grace, and faithfulness. To understand the Iona Community, it is critical to understand their historical context and their visions and practices of healing justice.

'Justice as Healing' is a chapter written by a former Leader of the Community, Kathy Galloway (Galloway 2000), outlining some of the Iona Community's vision and practice of healing justice. She suggests that, to be human in Jesus' way, is to practice a particular kind of healing justice. A justice that heals is about rediscovering what it is to be human. This rediscovering of our humanity Galloway sometimes calls 'learning our true names.' All members of the Iona Community do not use the language of healing justice, but many find it explains the heart of the Iona Community. Tom Gordon, an Iona Member, and hospice Chaplin, says the convergence of healing and justice lies at the heart of the Iona Community.

> If communities and the people within them are broken - by hopelessness and alienation and poverty and a lack of opportunity, etc., etc. - how can healing be found unless systems change, and justice is at the core. So, the two are inseparable, and, as such, gave the Iona Community its *raison d'etre*.

While some of the members report that the language of healing justice was new to them, they say it touched something core to the Iona Community, which is the view that justice, peace, and healing are inseparable.

The song quoted at the beginning of this chapter captures some key characteristics of the Community's under-standing of healing justice:

- Comes out of Christ and faithfulness to Christ.
- Is an expansive concept which does not fragment into many different realms.
- Is rediscovering wholeness within the embrace of Christ.
- Recognizes the special place of the broken in encountering God and understanding the world.
- Is about (re)establishing a particular kind of community.
- Is inclusion and acceptance.

Each of the characteristics requires some unpacking to understand the Iona Community's vision of healing justice.

Jesus Way of Love

Christ's is the world in which we move
Christ's are the folk we're summoned to love
Christ's is the voice that calls us to care
and Christ is the one who meets us there.

The Iona Community is a Christian community. For them, Christ is the beginning, the end, and the way. 'Christ's is the world in which we move.' For the Community, this means everything else flows out of and points towards Christ. In their Trinitarian theology, Christ, God, and the Spirit commingle such that to talk of Christ is to talk of God and Spirit. Drawing on their Celtic and Benedictine roots, they very often speak of God, Spirit, and Christ or Jesus.

The Leader of the Community told me they were a Christo-centric community. Then she changed her wording to a Jesus-centred community, suggesting the Community was focused on the life and humanity of Jesus. She was not denying the divinity of God nor making the divinity of Christ their focus. This is significant because the Iona Community is not held together by a common doctrine but a common practice. It is the practice of Jesus. As the song quoted in the opening of the chapter suggests, both the language of 'Christ' and of 'Jesus' is used, but in both cases, the focus is on the practice and life that flows out of Jesus and points towards Him.

The Iona Community's focus is not on *bringing Christ to* people or situations and trying to convince them to accept Christ. Rather, **the focus is on *discovering Christ in* the loving of those who have been marginalized.** 'Christ's is the voice that calls us to care, and Christ is the one who meets us there.' All people are Christ's and, in each person, particularly in those who are in mourning and those who are without resources, Christ is present. Seeing all people as Christ's or as created in the image of God leads some members of Iona to a non-violent stance, for to do violence to one of Christ's, created in God's image, is to do violence to God.

While the founder, George MacLeod, was clearly a pacifist and many in the community share his views, the Community has never adopted this stance of absolute pacifism. The Community understands itself as a Community committed to active non-violence, and this commitment is spelled out in multiple aspects of the Justice and Peace Commitment, which is binding on all the members. The Community also sees themselves as **nuclear pacifists.**

Since the face of Jesus is to be discerned in the poor, the hungry, the prisoners and the victims, social and political action could never be divorced from spirituality. Since the whole world is seen as Christ's, and therefore as holy, this view refuses to fragment or to polarize life into dichotomies. Life is always at the intersection of all things because, as the Bible declares, in Christ all things hold together (Colossians 1:17, NIV). In the Iona Community, worship, radical politics, and social action flow into and out of each other. Prayer and political action are both equal parts of Christian discipleship that inspired many of the first people who came to Iona for summer courses. Former leader Ferguson says they were trying to 'establish the view that political action for justice and peace was an imperative of the faith.'

One of the early leaders explained **the three-fold purpose of Iona** in these terms:

1. a call to discipleship that will lead to the peace of the world,
2. finding a way to meet the world's hunger, and
3. working for church unity.

The clear expectation is that Iona Community's mission is not for the conversion of the world (that the world might become Christian) but for the salvation of the world. The root of this word salvation is the same as the root of health and healing. In the Iona Community's context, salvation of the world is the healing of the world or the peace of the world.

The focus of the Iona Community is on **living a life that**

flows out of Christ and is a response to Him. Because they see the world as a sacrament of the presence of Christ, their life together is not based on separation but rather the co-existence of the sacred and the secular, work and worship, prayer and politics. This, too, is partly the basis of the Community's approach to healing. Ron Ferguson, former Leader of the Community, says, 'The Community's theology of healing was not one of magic intervention but of the corporate care of the Church in obedience to Jesus.' **They see healing justice as something God does. They are not the healers. They bring people to God through prayer and engaged action, but it is God who heals.**

Expanding the Circle of Connections

In the song above, those who are grieved by what we might call crime ('the women whom men have defiled') are grouped with those who are grieved by the loss of a child, and the hopeless, the lonely, the social misfits, the unemployed, the abused. Mainstream understandings of crime, harm, health, and social justice might deal with each of these in separate ways with different sets of experts to aid the process. However, the expansive view of healing in the Iona Community does not fragment or break things down in this manner.

Healing in the Iona Community is a broad concept somewhat similar to what some Aboriginal groups refer to as 'returning to balance.' It includes the healing of body, mind, and spirit of persons, and of the memories of communities and nations, as well as the healing of the earth. All are part of the ministry of healing, and they are all inextricably linked.

Concerning these intertwined linkages, Burgess writes,

> **I cannot pray for a young person in prison if I do not look for ways to relieve the boredom of unemployment, the pressure of advertising, the board and lodgings legislation that keeps him on the move, and the lure of drugs, which have combined to destroy his liberty.** I cannot pray for people who are poor in my community, or for that matter for people who are hungry, oppressed and poor anywhere else in the world if I do not challenge the way that my country's government spends its resources… If I am blind to the sources of injustice around me and divorce the needs of an individual from the pain of a whole community, my prayers for healing are nonsense and bear no resemblance to the good news of the gospel.

Thus, **prayer for healing** is always connected to the context of the wider world. As Iona Member and Dutch hospice chaplain, Desirée Van der Hijden put it: 'Illness may be caused by poverty, which makes praying for healing without working for justice rather useless in the long-term.'

In their resource book for the ministry of healing, *Praying for the Dawn*, Iona Community Member Burgess and Leader of the Community, Galloway, reflects this same expansive interconnectedness through their stories, services, and reflections. The stories represent this diversity, ranging from dealing with a young Northern Ireland woman's negative self-image to praying for the wholeness of the earth to the gradual healing of memories of a 63-year-old woman who had been raped three times.

The Community does not try to deal with each of the harms in precisely the same way. They are far too grounded in creation and the life of the housing projects of Glasgow to expect a one-size-fits-all response to healing. By holding this interrelatedness together in the context of a worshipping and learning community, they are trying to live out what Ron Ferguson calls 'a total gospel which held together worship and work, prayer and politics, personal and corporate healing, peace and justice.'

Kate McIlhagga tries to explain the Iona Community's perspective on the church's healing ministry.

   The healing ministry is first and foremost about justice and peace – about the healing of nations. But intertwined with that divine imperative is the healing of the individual, the healing of memory, of broken relationships.

Again, we see how this 'divine imperative' is intertwined in all of life. The health of the individual is not separate, in cause or effect, from the health of the larger community. The Iona Community focuses on healing prayer, but they refuse 'to hive off prayer and politics into separate compartments.'

An Iona Community publication describes the central theme of their healing ministry:

> It has always been a central theme of the healing ministry that we should look at the context in which illness and distress occur: so our ministry is as likely to take us into the realms of local and national politics, in an endeavour to change environments and policies which we believe to be responsible for individual illnesses and adversity of all sorts, as it is to be in direct contact with 'sick' people (The Iona Community 1996, p. 23).

One example that often gets repeated in the Iona Community is that **it is not enough to pray for someone dying of tuberculosis in the substandard housing in Glasgow.** One must also take political action in the matter of the housing project, which sets the environment within which one becomes more likely to contract tuberculosis. In the context of crime, this means the issues that lead an offender to offend must also be dealt with as part of a healing justice response.

Because 'Christ's is the world in which we move,' all things hold together in Christ. If all of life is woven together, then crime, harm, illness, distress, and war must be seen within the broad context. This is a vision and strategy of healing justice in the Iona Community.

Rediscovering Wholeness

To the lost Christ shows his face
to the unloved, he gives his embrace
to those who cry in pain or disgrace
Christ makes, with his friends, a touching place.

It follows from seeing life and healing within a broad concept that the object of healing is to return to wholeness. 'Healing is about the wholeness of people, 'at-one-ment' with themselves, their neighbors, their surroundings, and ultimately with God.' Returning to this wholeness is not about returning to the state of affairs before the particular harm happened. The wholeness of healing is the wholeness of coming into the embrace of Christ. It is a rediscovering of wholeness from the perspective of the One who created all things; therefore, the change required of healing justice is not limited to the mainstream boundaries of health, justice, and economics, private, or public. It also differs from many mainstream understandings of atonement that focus more on righting wrongs than the establishing of wholeness or at-one-ment. In fact, to address the brokenness of the world, the community saw the need to develop what some have called 'a holistic vision of political and theological justice.'

Another way of seeing this wholeness is to practice what Galloway calls 'Jesus' gospel of intrinsic worth.'

> ...in which all living things, including the earth itself, have innate value separate from and beyond their utility; in which the commodification, the selling, of all of life is resisted and reversed and in which justice is done. To be human in Jesus' way is to act justly.

Thus, the Iona Community's sense of healing justice is really a view of wholeness. Several Iona members told me this sense of justice involves responding to wrongs, but it moves beyond a reactive approach. Their holistic view of healing justice includes 'working for change and the renewal of systems so that people are sustained before they become broken by injustice, and, indeed, find their own methodologies to sustain themselves and heal others.' Addressing this same issue, another member explained how the vision of this justice extends to building compassionate communities.

" The vision certainly encompasses righting
wrongs but, like Jesus in his public ministry,
we are concerned with building community;
healing is about being brought back into
community, being cared for and being able to
love fully and freely without fear or abuse,
treating the earth as the precious resource
that we have been entrusted to care for.

So, the Iona Community's sense of justice is not merely a
reaction against injustice or a repairing-of-harm orientation. It is an orientation toward a deep sacred wholeness
that precedes and must inform any healing. Justice is a
wholeness found in the embrace of Christ.

Encountering God in the Broken

THE WAY into this wholeness is not through escaping
the pain of the world but through entering into the
mystery of suffering. In the mystery of suffering, one
begins to see the face of Christ.

HEALING JUSTICE in the Iona Community is entering the
mystery of suffering – the suffering of illness, the
suffering of systemic injustice, the suffering of

economies of war, and the suffering of inflicting harm. They believe these sufferings and injustices need to be central to the life of the church, but too often, the church avoids them or just talks without engaging in meaningful action. The purpose of the Iona Community is to support a network of people in ways the church has largely failed to do to help them to engage in encountering suffering and injustice with a vision and practice of a healing kind of justice. Engaging injustice has always been a central part of the witness of the Iona Community.

In the midst of this suffering, they expect to discover Christ and to discover a way to wholeness, which is healing justice.

Including and Accepting

To some people, the language of Christianity, which is so central to much of the discourse of the Iona Community, might seem exclusive and alienating. However, from the beginning, the Iona Community has tried to create space for those who have been marginalized to be included as friends or brothers and sisters. Because of their view of wholeness and their understandings of Christ, they do not draw sharp boundaries between Christian and non-Christian. All is one. Learning from **the Celtic view that God** is in all of life and in all of life is God, the Iona Community has developed a theology of inclusiveness. Nick Prance, an Iona Community Member and community mental health practitioner, explains how this vision-of-all prompts engaged action.

> I think if God is, God is one. We don't come into the world. We come out of it. It is this sense that prompts me to work towards a unified vision of humanity, which can hold different perspectives, but see them for what they are, simply perspectives.

They see this vision not just as for their community or the Christian church. They see it as a vision of healing justice for the whole world, including the land.

They believe that, by respecting all 'others' and accepting yourself, it is possible to create space for healing justice.

(Re)Establishing a Particular Kind of Community

The Iona Community was started, in part, to recover some of the communal dimensions of faith. They see Christianity, not as a private faith of individuals, but as a community-faith. The Rule mandates personal pieties, such as personal prayer and Bible reading, but the context is within a community vision of faith and life. In each case, in their island life, in the work of their experiments on the mainland, or in the life of their dispersed members, faith is about building a particular kind of community. For them, healing is about being brought back into community. To be community of a particular kind is both a vision and a practice of healing justice.

But what are the characteristics of this particular kind of community? First, as we have already seen, **a community is rooted in Christ for the sake of the world.** This is a worshipping, praying, learning community. It is also politically engaged, not afraid to speak truth to power.

Second, it is **a community willing to enter the brokenness of the world.** It is in the face of that brokenness they seek Christ and struggle together with the meaning of this brokenness in light of a vision of love. Such a community must be willing to risk, to act, and to experiment, which is to say, to learn through failing.

Third, **healing comes through living the questions and not accepting easy answers.** Therefore, communities must be of the type that creates space for wrestling with hard questions while, at the same time, coaching people to reject the easy answers.

Fourth, **such a community has a keen understanding of what they stand against and what they stand for.** As their booklet *What is the Iona Community?* explains, 'We hope to be not just a community which stands against injustice, oppression, and despair, but also a community which stands for hope, change, and celebration and affirmation of life together.'

Fifth, **such a community must be a sanctuary of love and of rediscovering identity.** In their words, 'This is the essence of the sanctuary – a place to feel loved, where you are valued for yourself and where your talents are welcome and useful – and if you thought you didn't have any, a place to discover that you have.'

What Healing Justice Is Not

I have tried to summarize the Iona Community's self-understanding of their approach to justice as healing. W. Graham Monteith, a member the community, took on a similar task to outline the Iona Community theology of healing embedded in the practice and liturgy of healing. He highlights several points that overlap with what I found:

- Healing and wholeness concern not only the individual but also the world.
- God through Jesus Christ is with us, and the world, in all our experience of life.
- Healing is sought through our own volition but granted by the will of God.
- An unquestioning faith is not a precondition of healing.
- God is always in solidarity with us.

Before we proceed to more of what healing justice looks like in the Iona Community, it is necessary to distinguish within the Iona Community what healing justice is not!

The Iona Community is quick to distinguish healing

from magic and a substitute for action. **Healing prayer** provides the motivation and vision for action. Healing is not about quick fixes, but about entering into the complex web of cosmic relationships and trying to find a way back to wholeness. Such a searching requires a long-term commitment to transformation, not an instant quick-fix expectation.

The Iona Community also distinguishes healing from medicine. The relationship between the two is complex. The way of healing is sometimes contrasted with the way of the surgeon, where the surgeon is depicted as adding more harm by cutting the body, and healing is described as gently tending the body, so it has space to heal itself and return to wholeness. Such tending, according to Galloway, includes 'prayer, deep attentiveness to the suffering of others but also to their giftedness.' There is an implied contrast with a medical model, which tends to be more intrusive, focusing exclusively on the material and driven by an expert who has little or no awareness of the giftedness of the one she is treating.

In a similar vein Ferguson, past Leader of the Community, claims the dominant modern scientific approach to life and medicine has also been

 ...devastating for health. Along with science generally, it has had spectacular successes, but it has led inexorably to 'magic bullet' medicine, where the doctor prescribes a drug to deal with symptoms. The whole person is

missing. Everything is cast into the problem/solution mold.

They argue that science is more likely to lead to a magical pill mentality than the kind of prayerful approach they are seeking to cultivate.

However, it would be wrong to assume the Iona Community is against the medical health discipline. Their Worship Book says both medicine and healing are gifts and work well together. Former leader Graeme Brown states the relationship this way: 'The Iona Community affirms the Health Service but is critical of those who assume that medicines alone are required for wholeness.' Monteith reports that many Iona members are engaged in the healing profession, and their engaging in both healing and medicine has been mutually beneficial.

The Iona Community's approach to healing justice is in contrast with the modern scientific vision, but they do not function in isolation, using only their approach to the exclusion of all others. An example of this is that healing prayer is not offered instead of other action but precisely to spark prayerfully engaged action. Their expansive approach to wholeness and to expecting Christ in the stranger leads them to expect to find giftedness wherever they look, including medicine.

Justice and Peace Commitment

Behind the Iona Community's practice of healing justice is the **Justice and Peace Commitment of the Community.** As part of their Rule, all members agree to practice this commitment in who they are, what they do, and what they don't do. It is quoted here at length because of its centrality in the practice of healing justice in the Iona Community.

 Justice and Peace Commitment:

We believe:

1. that the Gospel commands us to seek peace founded on justice and that costly reconciliation is at the heart of the Gospel;

2. that work for justice, peace and an equitable society is a matter of extreme urgency;

3. that God has given us partnership as stewards of creation and that we have a responsibility to live in a right relationship with the whole of God's creation;

4. that, handled with integrity, creation can provide for the needs of all, but not for the greed which leads to injustice and inequality, and endangers life on earth;

5. that everyone should have the quality and

dignity of a full life that requires adequate physical, social and political opportunity, without the oppression of poverty, injustice, and fear;

6. that social and political action leading to justice for all people and encouraged by prayer and discussion is a vital work of the Church at all levels;

7. that the use or threatened use of nuclear and other weapons of mass destruction is theologically and morally indefensible and that opposition to their existence is an imperative of the Christian faith.

As Members and Family Groups we will:

8. engage in forms of political witness and action, prayerfully and thoughtfully, to promote just and peaceful social, political and economic structures;

9. work for a British policy of renunciation of all weapons of mass destruction and for the encouragement of other nations, individually or collectively, to do the same;

10. celebrate human diversity and actively work to combat discrimination on grounds of age, color, disability, mental wellbeing, differing ability, gender, color, race, ethnic

and cultural background, sexual orientation or religion;

11. work for the establishment of the United Nations Organization as the principal organ of international reconciliation and security, in place of military alliances;

12. support and promote research and education into non-violent ways of achieving justice, peace and a sustainable global society;

13. work for reconciliation within and among nations by international sharing and exchange of experience and people, with particular concern for politically and economically oppressed nations.

It is the commitment of each member, with support from family groups and the larger Iona Community network, to figure out how to practice these commitments within their own life and location. Just how that is done varies to a considerable degree within the membership. However, there are some practices that seem quite common among the Iona Community.

I will highlight seven aspects of how the Iona Community practices healing justice.

Living Together

I have briefly outlined one practice of healing justice in the Iona Community – to live in community together. A whole book could be devoted to describing the significance of this to healing justice. Such a book would, no doubt, have to consider the role of feasting and celebrating together, sharing in the work of basic survival, struggling together, responding to change, exercises of leadership, decision-making processes, processes of letting go, processes of inspiration and teaching and more.

Modelling Life

Most of the members I talked to spoke of trying to model a positive way of justice in their lifestyle. Kathy Galloway calls this the 'practice (of) voluntary self-limitation to model the kind of political and cultural life that is hoped for.' Galloway sees self-limitation needed in areas of consumerism, cultural and spiritual imperialism, and in forced or manipulated proselytism. In fact, she says that our inability to live self-limited lives leads to wars, pandemics, structural inequalities, and ecological holocaust. Members talked to me about trying to live simply, to decrease dependency on oil by purchasing locally, to grow their own food, and to purchase environmentally friendly products. They spoke of trying to address some of the global inequalities by **buying Fair Trade products** and **eating mostly vegetarian foods**.

The island centers also model this kind of healing justice. Raising environmental issues to do with the sustainable care of the earth is a long-standing tradition in the Iona Community, going back at least into the 1950s.

It seems that members of the Iona Community model healing justice relationships in the kinds of jobs or careers they vocation. Many of them work in some helping or advocating role. Ronald Ferguson's history of Iona Community closes with many stories of how Iona members have tried, and are trying, to live out this vision of justice as healing in their lives and work. One such story is that of Reverend Walter Fyfe, who was concerned that unemployed and poorly paid people needed more power over the direction of their lives. His work was to help train groups to establish credit unions and other money-borrowing schemes. His goal was that they could cut their dependence on loan sharks while creating local power that could be used to tackle other issues. Other members told me about working at, and advocating for, a host of other issues, a sampling of which includes: anti-discrimination against gay, lesbian and transgendered people; the anti-apartheid movement; the anti-nuclear movement; international relief work; life story work with *Alzheimer's Society; political election campaigns; and interfaith dialogue.*

The Iona Community also seems to value thoughtful reflections. Many members work to advocate the kind of life they hope for by writing books, songs, and liturgies around peace and justice issues.

Engaging Injustice and Sometimes Breaking the Law

The Iona Community encourages their members to stand up to injustices where they are found. Sometimes, this even means breaking the law where they perceive the law to be unjust. An example of this would be their work against the **nuclear Trident defense plan**. Some members used non-violent direct action to try to resist these initiatives and to articulate a more healing and just alternative. For example, some Iona Community members were arrested for lying down in front of traffic outside the location where the Trident nuclear weapons are held. Another member, together with others, destroyed some equipment pertaining to the Trident program and then turned themselves in and made their arguments through the court system.

Restoring Harms

The Iona Community believes restoration of harms can happen through 'respectful dialogue of equals which builds common ground and relationships of friendship while dispelling ignorance and healing the memory of past divisions.' When harms arise within the Community, they try to follow such a process. However, they were quick to note that the work of responding wisely to harm must begin long before the harm takes place. Building a community of trust, unity, compassion, and common vision before harms create the space to respond in healing ways. However, once harm has happened,

they seem to follow some clear but unwritten
procedures.

- **Recognize brokenness.** Brokenness happens
  and, if it does not have space to surface
  constructively, it only becomes more
  destructive.
- **Listen to the story and seek to understand.**
- **Find others in the community to help** if those
  in conflict get stuck. Others could help as
  trainers or as facilitators.
- **Seek forgiveness, if appropriate, and try to
  make things right as much as people are able.**
  This is done as a direct encounter between the
  people who have experienced this harm and,
  sometimes, with the presence of a supporting
  community.
- **Work for contexts where harming doesn't
  happen so easily.** Trying to address the broader
  context is one of the hallmarks of the Iona
  Community's approach to harm, whether it is
  the harm between persons or the harm of unjust
  global structures.

Through their **youth department**, the Iona Community
has a longstanding relationship with the Polmont Young
Offender Institute. Members have been visiting those
who are incarcerated, and those incarcerated have been
coming to the Iona Community Camas centers to experience a simple lifestyle in tune with the local environ-

ment. Camas is a center on the coast of the Isle of Mull accessible only by walking a couple of miles. It has little electricity and groups have to work together to feed each other and help each other to survive. Iona Community members have reported seeing huge changes within the young people who had been incarcerated and between them and the adult staff who accompanied them.

The youth department engages in a program that tries to apply some of these insights of healing justice to youth who have been convicted of a crime. This is called **Project Jacob (Scotland)**, which is a partnership between the Iona Community, Project Scotland, the Church of Scotland, Time for God, and Project Jacob England. They work with young people aged 16-25 who are completing their sentences at Scotland's Polmont Young Offender Institute.

The young people are given the opportunity to change their lifestyle as a means of creating the kind of environments that lead to healing justice, rather than injustice. By working through the Polmont Institute chaplain, who is an Associate Member of the Iona Community, young people can apply for Project Jacob. In this program, young people are given 'full-time volunteer work, supported accommodation, individual pastoral care, and support and befriending.' Of the first twelve Scottish young people who participated in the pilot project of this program, none has re-offended. The idea is to help young people to move into a healthy lifestyle, to gain practical experience and confidence, and to earn positive references.

The Iona Community is working in Glasgow and Edinburgh to partner with housing associations. The Iona Community shares risk by taking out a tenancy agreement with the housing association on behalf of the young person. Through working with the young people for three months to two years and through volunteer mentoring and the support of a care worker, they try to cultivate conditions of friendship and support, so the young people can integrate back into the community in healthy ways.

The longstanding youth work in Camas with young offenders from Polmont Institution and the Jacob Project are two examples of how the Iona Community works within the area of crime. A third is the number of community members who have become chaplains of prisons. A fourth is the Community's work in the 1960s, when they were part of the lobbying that helped to **abolish the death penalty**. The Iona Community works within the criminal justice system but tries to bring aspects of humanization and restorative justice to their relationships with those called offenders.

Praying for Healing

George MacLeod, the founding Leader of the Community, called on the community to work at healing by intercession and **laying-on of hands. Intercessory prayer** is part of the healing prayer service that has been part of the Iona Community's witness for over sixty years. On Tuesday evening, people on the Isle of Iona are invited to gather in the Abbey for a **Service of Prayer and Healing.**

The service has always given participants the opportunity to place before God people with illnesses, situations with discord, and nations broken by strife. Prayer requests are received from people who are visitors to the community on Iona and by letter and telephone from many parts of the world. A list of requests is created to be used during the service and then left in St. Columba's Chapel until the following service. Because the prayer requests are about brokenness, in particular, people, as well as particular situations in the world, the services focus mainly on physical wellbeing, but also take note of political and social aspects of a situation and walking with the poor.

The Service of Prayer for Healing often opens with this welcome and opening response:

Leader: We gather here in your presence God,

ALL: IN OUR NEED AND BRINGING WITH US THE NEEDS OF THE WORLD.

Leader: We come to you, for you come to us in Jesus

ALL: AND YOU KNOW BY

EXPERIENCE WHAT HUMAN LIFE IS LIKE

Leader: We come with our faith and with our doubts;

ALL: WE COME WITH OUR HOPES AND WITH OUR FEARS.

Leader: We come as we are because it is God who invites us to come,

ALL: AND GOD HAS PROMISED NEVER TO TURN US AWAY

After a song (like the one quoted in the opening of this chapter) and some Scripture reading, the prayers of intercession are offered. Each person or situation is mentioned by name but without much detail. It is as if mentioning them in this context is enough.

The Iona Prayer Circle functions outside of the prayer service but also participates in the work of intercession. This work is regarded as so significant that the Prayer Circle secretary is a permanent appointment within the community. The Prayer List used by them is 'circulated throughout the UK and to the circle of intercessors, living all over the world.'

Part of the Rule that members of Iona agree to is to pray regularly and frequently for each other. This, too, is part of intercessory prayer. An annual prayer guidebook is created for members, which includes prayer for each member by name once a month on a particular day. Thus, daily intercessory prayer is also part of the Rule of the Iona Community members.

In the Service of Prayer for Healing, immediately following the prayers of intercession is the laying-on of hands.

Ruth Burgess explains the laying-on of hands.

> What happens is that those asking for prayer will come and kneel in a circle on cushions laid out in a space in the middle of the church, and others will stand beside them. When the worship leaders pray for an individual, they will place their hands on the individual's head, and at the same time, those nearest the person being prayed for will put a hand on the person's shoulder or arm. A prayer is then said for the person, worship leaders and congregation saying the words together, often:
>
> *Spirit of the living God, present with us now,*
>
> *Enter you, body, mind, and spirit, and heal you of all that harms you.*
>
> *In Jesus name, amen.*
>
> Often those not near enough to touch the person being prayed for will put a hand on the shoulder of the person standing nearest to

them, as a way of being physically involved in the prayer. When all those kneeling have been prayed for, they stand up and let others take their place. They can choose to return to their seats or remain as part of the group sharing the laying-on of hands.

Margaret Stewart, medical doctor, and minister spoke in the introduction to a healing service concerning the laying-on of hands:

66 We come forward with concern for our lack of wholeness, for family and friends, for broken community and by our action, in asking and accepting the hands of the people who travel alongside us tonight we open ourselves to the power of the Spirit. Such can energize the healing process present in our bodies, our minds, and our spirits.

Often this laying-on of hands will happen while a song is sung. The Service of Prayer for Healing then ends with a closing prayer and benediction.

Laying-on of hands is not exercised by one person but by the whole community as they bring a person or situation to the healing attention of God. Typically, this laying-on of hands occurs within a healing prayer service. Ruth Burgess wrote part of the liturgy for this service. She explains how she sees the role of community in healing.

> My perception of what we do is that we create a space for God to act. This is what worship is… bringing people into an awareness of God's presence and action. It is not us that create energy. We create context. The action comes from God. It can come through us but does not originate in us, and we cannot 'make' anything happens. We ask God to act.

Another context of prayer is **the Daily Office**, which all members follow. The Daily Office is an annual guide for Iona members, as each day, a different member is prayed for.

Learning from the 'Other'

Kathy Galloway explains that justice as healing is a justice that includes learning 'from the justice and peacemakers of other faiths, and from artists, ecologists and community activists among others.' The Iona Community has learned from their interdenominational heritage that they need to be open and attentive to others. They must seek justice, not just within the church, but also by learning from a variety of others. Galloway says these others include both neighbor and enemy. They must seek security by establishing friendships and through seeking the security of others rather than their insecurity. The Iona Community and its members are quite active in interfaith relations as they take the opportunity to participate in and to host forums to explore these themes.

Engaging Accountability

Members reported their practice of healing justice included being accountable for their finances and their time. Such accountability is indicated in the second and third items of the Community's Rule. Members meet together in **Family Groups** for support, encouragement, and accountability. These Family Groups are one of the places members are challenged and supported to live out the **Justice and Peace Commitment**. Members are encouraged to account for 90% of their disposable income. It is expected that they tithe, some of their donation going to the Iona Community, some to the church, and some to charities the member supports. Graeme Brown, former Leader of the Community, summarized to me how this practice is experienced in the community:

> This kind of transparency is quite a demanding and, at times, painful thing. We tend not to be very hard on one another, but we do believe that this kind of exercise is intrinsic to our personal and corporate search for justice.

By being accountable for their time and money, they create an environment that supports innovative experiments in living and modeling their lives, based on their best insights so far into what healing justice looks like in practice.

The goal is to be purposeful in every aspect of how life is lived. How we spend our money and time marks how we move through the world. The Iona Community seems to believe we can move through the world in violent and destructive ways or just and peaceful ways. By calling people to follow the rules of accountability for time and money, the Community is trying to offer its members support and encouragement to move through the world in more just, peaceful, and healing ways.

In some ways, the practices of healing justice in the Iona Community are as diverse as its members, each one embodying the vision in different ways and different places. In the preceding section, I have tried to highlight some of the common features of that practice. But what inspires or sustains such a vision of justice? That is the subject of the next section.

How does the Iona Community identify the various conditions and factors, the cultural dynamics, which sustain their vision of justice as healing? As with each of the communities examined here, none of these factors independently stand on their own. Each dynamic is connected to and informed by the others. It is better to imagine these as a web of dynamics than a list of ingredients.

Cultivating Commons

Healing justice is sustained by a sense of a community holding common directions, principles, and tasks. For the Iona Community, the common direction is largely summed up in the Peace and Justice Commitment. One member called the common direction the Kingdom of God. Another called it a commitment to a radical under-standing of the gospel. Their five-fold Rule offers a prac-tice that all community members agree to pursue. These common practices, over time, create both the cohesion and tensions of belonging to a diverse group. When it is working, the practice of the Rule creates the trust and openness required to pursue justice as healing. Healing justice is sustained by a shared vision.

The Iona Community believes that ideas are not enough. They believe that ideas must be embodied in a living community before they can be of service. This view is sometimes called incarnation about how God became flesh in the person Jesus or the world. Jesus is not seen as some distant ideal but as a way of embodying the love of God in the midst of the varying social, political, and material dynamics of the day. This embodying of love at every stage is the vision, the means, and end of ministry of the Iona Community.

The founding Leader of the Iona Community, George MacLeod, stressed this focus on engaged love by focusing on common tasks. In his words, 'A compelling common task alone creates community.' This initial task was the rebuilding of the Abbey and the engaging of the political-theological imagination of the workers. The second Leader of the Community, Ian Reid, also affirmed their task was the rebuilding of people and relationships. A ministry of friendship has been a defining characteristic of the Iona Community since the very early days. Kathy Galloway claims the Iona Community is not sustained through theories or commandments but something like the urge to friendship.

> The impetus to do this hard and often unpopular work (of justice as healing) does not come from theories or 'thou shalts.' It comes, like the urge to friendship, from our desire for what is lively, vivid, life-enhancing, for freedom and laughter, for all the things we give and receive in friendship.

Healing justice is sustained by a common direction and task that is relational, spiritual, and political. The Rule calls on members to be engaged outside their own Community in the task of building and rebuilding a politics of love in the world.

Reading Bible, Praying and Worshipping

The Iona Community members were very clear that their orientation to a justice that heals is sustained by practices of **Bible reading**, prayer, liturgy, and worship. Their first Rule has to do with daily prayer and regular and frequent

Bible reading. The knowledge that someone is praying for you and that you need to pray for others helps to sustain them in their work for peace and justice.

They believe there is a link between these practices of Christian faith and healing justice in the world. The Iona Deputy Leader of 17 years, Ralph Morton, claims there is a direct link between Christian discipleship and the peace of the world. Moreover, he claims that finding 'anew the way of discipleship' is the beginning place of all other action.

> The first thing that is demanded of the followers of Jesus Christ is that they find anew the way of discipleship for men in the world today. This is the first demand because without it we can never begin and therefore never do anything else... It may seem ridiculous to link such a seemingly useless thing as this with so terrifying a problem as the peace of the world. But it is the only thing we have to offer. It is the only way by which the peace of the world will be assured.

In Morton's perspective, the Iona Community cannot begin to contribute towards the peace of the world directly. It can do so only by looking again at what it means to be a follower of Jesus Christ. This Christ that the Iona Community must follow cannot be reduced to principles, values, or universal cultural dynamics. The

Community will need to find its direction by seeking ways of following Jesus, ways that perhaps have been forgotten and need to be revived, or perhaps new ways that are responsive to the world today.

The Iona Community is quick to recognize how Christians have been embroiled in colonialization, genocide, and capitalistic empire building. While the Christian Right is perhaps the most well-known current movement trying to bring Christian piety and politics together, the Iona Community is articulating a very different alternative. For them, the solution is in taking Jesus more seriously. It is their prayer, Bible reading, and worship that lead them to engage in healing kinds of justice. This radical particularity, they believe, equips them to be a gift for the world and to connect respectfully and participate with those who have different religious beliefs.

Facing Suffering

One of the most significant factors in sustaining healing justice in the Iona Community is that they **choose to stand near the disadvantaged.** The Iona Community believes where it stands will enlighten what it thinks. The Community stands with one foot on an island of great beauty and the other in the heart of the inner city. In both places, they encounter the beauty and the suffering of the world. It is what Iona Member Tom Gordon calls a focus on reality.

66 What, I believe, has sustained the Iona Community, through changing generations and membership, is its focus on reality. It seeks not to stand apart but to engage with real issues and real people. This is not to say that it has now, or ever has had all the answers. But it faces real and painful issues honestly and is prepared to take a stand on what is important.

Another member of the Iona Community explains how facing the suffering of the world sparks the practice of healing justice.

66 The most significant impetus for the sustained commitment to healing justice is the state of the world in which we live. It was the needs of the developing world which drew me into Christian education in Africa. It was the starvation of the people of Biafra which drew me into relief work. It was the oppression of black people in South Africa which drew me to share in theological education there and then into the anti-apartheid struggle. In all of these areas, there were members of the Iona Community there before me.

Facing the suffering of the world through the eyes of

Christ leads members of the Iona Community to engage more deeply with the world.

Standing Near Creation

Drawing on the Celtic insistence that all life is sacred, the Iona Community is sustained by standing near creation. One member said Creation is an incarnation and emanation. God's creation flows out of God and gives body to the character of God. By standing near and recognizing the sacredness of creation, you touch God, and this transforms your way of living. This view of the sacredness of all life creates what Kathy Galloway calls a 'self-disciplined ethos of reverence and respect for cultural, spiritual and bio-diversity alike....'

Ferguson argues the survival of the planet is dependent on the notion of **sacramental reverence**, replacing notions of dominance and exploitation.

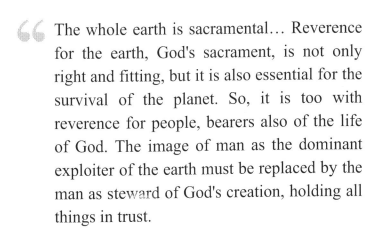

> The whole earth is sacramental... Reverence for the earth, God's sacrament, is not only right and fitting, but it is also essential for the survival of the planet. So, it is too with reverence for people, bearers also of the life of God. The image of man as the dominant exploiter of the earth must be replaced by the man as steward of God's creation, holding all things in trust.

The Iona Community today tends not to use exclusive male language to refer to all of humanity. Because including those who have been marginalized is a key theme of the community, it is important to them to avoid exclusive male language. Healing justice is sustained by seeing the sacredness of all of life, all of creation.

Engaging Your Own Brokenness and Complicity

In the Iona Community, healing justice is sustained by engaging your own brokenness and your complicity in the brokenness of the world.

> But for many of us, healing only begins when we recognize our own complicity, not only as victims, but also as perpetrators, and we go at last to all those who suffered for us and ask to be received back. In some deep sense, those who died were the random victims of all of us who survived. And those who mourn, mourn for all of us.

Duncan Morrow was speaking about how their lens of healing justice interprets the situation in Northern Ireland. He captures some factors that seem to sustain healing justice in the Iona Community. Healing justice does not come from distant experts. It comes from those who are complicit in the wrongs of the world but are trying to find a path of healing. It comes, not from those who have the perfect plan for restoration, but from those who are willing to confess their own brokenness. The Iona Community has traditionally seen itself as a servant of the church at large. They are quick to remember that 'Christianity itself needs to be healed.' One example of this is the **daily morning prayer**, which includes a section on confession. Such a focus could nurture a paralysis of guilt, but here it seems to sustain a way of being engaged in healing of others as you are in the process of healing. It is the willingness to engage your own brokenness that helps to sustain healing justice.

Living as a Collective

The Iona Community was established, in part, to experiment with how living in a community might sustain a different vision of being the church in the world. Through sixty plus years of experiment, they are convinced that a supportive community is needed to sustain their life and vision, but such a community is not an end in itself. As one member told me, they try to offer an alternative to two flawed models of the church: the church as the one-to-one relationship with God (the liberal individualist model) and the church as the self-serving and self-perpetuating institution (the conservative model). Each model has difficulty sustaining healing justice, the individualist model because it cannot see beyond the individual; the conservative model as it cannot see beyond itself. Being engaged as a community is about discovering and responding to Christ in the world. When healthy, this community sees beyond itself, even to the point of letting itself die. This community, in the Iona Community's understanding, is there for the good of the world, to bring healing, justice, and peace.

Supporting Each Other

The Iona Community continues today as a support network for Christians engaged in peace and justice activities that cannot find support within the traditional church structure. One aspect of this support is account-ability, the fifth and last rule of the community. Numerous members told me that what sustained their practice of healing justice was the support and loving challenges they received from the community through monthly Family Groups, **Community Week**, plenary meetings, and through prayers.

Being a Movement

The Iona Community believes that, to sustain their prac-tices of healing justice, they must organize as a move-ment or an organism, rather than an institution. To live as a movement means a wide range of things: to maintain light structures; to be attentive to the vision, stimulus and change that young people bring; to let some things die; to see the community as scaffolding rather than as building; to listen to and be surprised by other people's ideas and stories; to accept change; and to take risks.

The Iona Community does not see healing justice as

something that can be institutionalized. They believe the less institutionalized and geared towards permanence they are, the more space they have to risk and explore the kinds of relationships that come out of a justice that heals.

Listening to the Stories of Those Who Have Gone Before

One feature that surfaced in several interviews as a sustaining factor was listening to the stories of other members of the Iona Community. Just hearing the stories of what others have done and are doing inspires them to action. This seems to be the primary purpose of the community's bi-monthly magazine, *The Coracle*, and many of the books published by the Iona Community's publishing house, **Wild Goose Publications**. Listening to the stories of others doing the work of healing justice seems to spark the courage and imagination necessary to engage injustice in your own context.

Nurturing Deep Roots

The Iona Community believes a charity model of aid is insufficient to sustain a justice that heals. The focus of international peace needs to shift from 'focusing on quick fixes, and emergency aid, (to focusing on the) issue of war on want,' as former leader Ferguson puts it. It is **the greed of the world that must be addressed** through forms of decreasing want and increasing sharing.

What sustains their view of justice is a desire to move beneath the symptoms and crisis and to find paths of healing grounded in the life of the world and therefore in the reverent respect for all of life. The grounding in life is what they see as having sustained their commitment to healing.

In the various experiments of faith in inner-city Glasgow and around the world, the Iona Community has tried to nurture indigenous expressions of faith. Leader Ferguson puts it this way:

> The goal of the small and vulnerable churches in the housing schemes and inner-city areas is to struggle to form indigenous expressions of faith over against a paternalistic, dominant Church...

The refusal to impose a system on everyone helps to create space for the rise of indigenous or locally-rooted expressions of healing justice. This desire for local expressions of faith and life came out as a strong theme in my interviews.

A tension or inconsistency emerges here. Within the Iona Community's project to nurture meaningful worship, they have collected songs from around the world and written many of their own, sometimes following local folk songs. They have also written many dramas and liturgies. As these materials are made available through the worship resource group and publishing arm, they have become an export commodity and are used around the world. Some churches depend more on importing the resources of the Iona Community than on creating their own. However, the goal of the Iona Community is not for other groups to become like them but rather that peace, justice, and healing are nurtured and supported in local ways by local people.

Critical Solidarity

The Iona Community engages in political debate with the leaders of the day. In the last election in Scotland, Iona Members or Associates ran for five different parties. However, they do so from the standpoint of critical solidarity. In the Iona context, the frame is not the usual separation of church and state, nor is it an agenda for a neo-Christendom. They seem to believe the church is at its best when it is 'radical, freewheeling, prophetic, refusing to bend the knee. When it degenerates into a prudential buttress for the powers-that-be, it sells Jesus down the river.' Christians need to have the ability to challenge and to support the state to act in just ways.

In the view of the Iona Community, Christians must have the capacity to break the laws of the state if they are seen as unjust. Some Iona members have spent time in jail because of what they see as witnessing against the unjust ways of the state. There is an important distinction being made here. The church ceases to be a sustaining force for healing justice when it becomes an unconditional buttress to the powers-that-be.

The dynamics that sustain healing justice approaches in the Iona Community do not function in isolation. Each dynamic is interconnected with the others, all functioning together to help support a justice that heals. To understand their approach better, it is also necessary to understand what they believe acts as a barrier to healing justice.

Barriers To Healing Justice

In my dialogues with members of the Iona Community, I got a wide range of responses concerning what functions as a barrier to healing justice. Again, I have only listed ideas that surfaced from more than one source. If members of the Iona Community were brought together to dialogue on this topic, they would likely have a much longer and more in-depth list.

Prejudices, Beliefs, and Mistrusts

The Iona Community believes barriers to healing justice arise internally, sometimes even within those individuals seeking such a justice. Members told me stories of when thinking one owned the truth or mistrusting difference in others created huge barriers between people. One member told of how the prejudices of a member damaged the relationships with a group the community was trying to reach out to and thereby set back relationships and opportunities to enhance healing justice. A barrier to healing justice may come from within, among its advocates.

Church as Part of Injustice

Although many members of the Iona Community work within the church, the church is also seen as potentially one of the barriers to healing justice. They listed many ways the church has been and continues to be involved with injustice rather than healing justice. Some of the particular issues were excluding gay and lesbian couples from leadership roles in the Church, excluding women from the church, and teaching people that sickness is a result of lack of faith. Christian theology and teaching that focuses on 'personally being right with God' as the only item of concern were also used to illustrate how sometimes the theology of churches blinds them to seeing their own systems and structures that also need transforming and reconciling.

Power Struggles and the Desire to Impose

It seems that hierarchical power structures act as barriers to healing justice. The desire to win or to impose one system, idea, or ethos on everyone was identified as a barrier to the creation of communities of healing justice. Similarly, patriarchal power structures were identified as a barrier. Both patriarchal and hierarchical power was seen to limit risk-taking, creativity, and the ability to let go, factors seen as necessary components of a community committed to healing justice.

Mainstream Political Systems

Many features of mainstream political systems were highlighted as creating barriers to healing justice. I think the focus on mainstream systems came, in part, from their relative influence but also from the desire to be accountable for one's own system. The significant apathy and disillusionment with politics among the general population was highlighted as a symptom of a system not working. Healing justice tends to be grassroots by nature, and in mainstream political systems, it is inhibited by the distance between those in power and those in real life. The tradition of separating government and religion was also identified as a barrier. Because the Iona Community comes at healing justice through a politics modeled after the life and teachings of Jesus, separation of church and state makes little sense to them. When church is ruled out of the public sphere and is regarded as a private spiritual matter, a barrier to healing justice arises. A justice that heals is interested in spiritual and physical, the political and the personal, the wound and the structures and systems that surround it. Mainstream politics sometimes leave little room for this kind of expansive view of justice and therefore can act as a barrier to it.

Capitalism, the Division between Rich and Poor and the Fear of Loss

Economic and political theories, like capitalism, were identified as key barriers to healing justice. In part, this is because Community members believe that such structures are designed to keep people poor and uneducated. Those in the West tend to live at ecologically and culturally unsustainable levels. Even within the West, the gap between rich and poor continues to grow. Members of the Iona Community, by and large, self-identify themselves as the rich, relative to the majority of the world. They recognize that the healing of injustices around the world would require different economic systems and ways of living, especially for the rich. A barrier to such change is the fear of loss of wealth, power, and control. The rich would have to move out of their comfort zones, and this is one of the major barriers to healing justice.

Desire for Permanence

The desire to keep organizations and structures alive forever is another part of what keeps healing justice from flourishing. When corporate identities outlive their purpose, they tend to institutionalize, bureaucratize, and move into a replication mode. Under these conditions, healing justice struggles. Communities that support healing justice need space for change, transformation, the dying of old-fashioned ways, and birthing of new ideas. The institutional desire for permanence acts as a barrier to healing justice.

Final Words

I have tried to share the story of the Iona Community from the perspective of healing justice. It is an attempt to tell the story of how they understand and approach healing justice. For the Iona Community, healing justice comes out of their faith orientation but pushes them to work in solidarity with many people who do not share that faith orientation. A defining feature of their approach is to focus on the personal, the structural, and the spiritual as if they are one. This orientation has taken them from the inner city to global politics, from disease to the problems of capitalism, from crime to issues of poverty and greed. Here, healing justice moves freely between personal episodes and structural change. At each step along the path of healing justice, the Iona Community has tried to recognize the sacredness of all creation such that healing justice becomes finding your humanity, recognizing the image of God in others, listening to and caring for creation, and finding ways to embrace those on the fringes.

Chapter 5 - Listening to the Stories: What Kind of Love and Wisdom is This?

Reconciliation

We are waking up to our history
from a forced slumber
We are breathing it into our lungs
so it will be part of us again
It will make us angry at first
because we will see how much you stole from us
and for how long you watched us suffer
we will see how you see us
and how when we copied your ways
we killed our own.

We will cry and cry and cry
because we can never be the same again
But we will go home to cry

and we will see ourselves in this huge mess
and we will gently whisper the circle back
and it will be old and it will be new.

Then we will breathe our history back to you
you will feel how strong and alive it is
and you will feel yourself become a part of it
And it will shock you at first
because it is too big to see all at once
and you won't want to believe it
you will see how you see us
and all the disaster in your ways
how much we lost.

And you will cry and cry and cry
because we can never be the same again
But we will cry with you
and we will see ourselves in this huge mess
and we will gently whisper the circle back
and it will be old and it will be new
(Tabobondung 2002).

This poem by a Canadian Aboriginal author highlights some of the ways healing justice might be taken seriously. The poem opens the book, *Nation to Nation: Aboriginal Sovereignty and the Future of Canada*. It addresses the process by which nation to nation dialogue might evolve between First Nations and Canada. To me, it highlights many aspects of healing justice and my journey into healing justice.

Taking healing justice seriously requires creating places where communities can 'wake up to our history, from a forced slumber.' Aboriginal peoples are starting to wake up and see how colonialization, assimilation, and the resource demands of capitalism have forced them into a deep slumber. They have forgotten who they are. They have lost the ways they traditionally used to survive, heal, adapt, and flourish. When forced to copy foreign ways, it killed their own. And now, waking up is not easy. It is an experience of anger, injustice, and shock. But the response is not to attack or even to transform the state that forced this slumber. Their response is to go home, to cry together, and to learn to whisper the circle back. The Hollow Water community's story is surely such a story. Their goal is not to return to some golden age in the past but to create the space to engage such that, 'it will be old and it will be new.'

As Aboriginal people rediscover who they are, they are discovering many beautiful and valuable resources within their culture and traditions. Some have articulated this rediscovery as healing justice.

But it is not just Aboriginal people who are waking up from a forced slumber. We see in Plum Village a community organized in such a way that people might wake up, be mindful, and engage the whole world with compassion. Here, the forced slumber comes in part through the trauma of the Vietnam War and, in part, through the pressures of modern society. They, too, speak of needing to rediscover one's true identity, of needing to 'breathe it into our lungs,' and of learning to go back home to gently whisper the circle back. They recognize that, in our world, it is often easier to live in forgetfulness than mindfulness. They try to identify practices that can sustain an awakened, mindful, and engaged way of being.

In the Iona Community, we also see this sense of waking up from a forced slumber, a slumber brought about by industrialization and by theologies that separate spiritual from political and action for justice from the prayers of the people. They, too, speak of needing to learn their true names, about seeing how they are connected to the world, and about learning to start with the innate goodness of all creation rather than the original sinfulness of human beings.

In these communities, healing justice is discovered through a process of going home to weep together. Taking healing justice seriously for them is not first and foremost about adapting to the state system. Taking healing justice seriously is first about finding spaces for communities to wake up, to see the ways they have been forced asleep, to feel how much they have lost, and to learn that copying foreign ways all too often kills local ways. The communities in this study have created and are creating such space.

According to the poem, change to the larger society comes as:

we will breathe our history back to you
you will feel how strong and alive it is
and you will feel yourself become a part of it.

For me, this was what happened by traveling between these communities. They breathed their history into me, and I could feel how alive it was, and I could feel myself becoming a part of it. However, learning this new geography of healing justice is not easy. I saw that modern communities around the world could respond to harms, not with punishment, blame, and fear, but with trying to offer help, healing, and transformation. I found a sense of justice, not rooted in administering pain, but in cultivating joy. I found that healing justice was not a romantic aspiration but was a practical reality practiced by diverse communities around the world. Soon, hard questions about my own traditions emerged or, as the poem says: 'you will see how you see us, and all the disaster in your ways.'

Have the Western state systems of justice forced us into a slumber? Not just Aboriginal people, but all people. As we have copied colonializing ways, did it kill our own? Do we have a history, an identity, a people that we can go back home to and learn to cry together and to gently whisper the circle back? What might it look like for different nations to come together to see ourselves in this huge mess and to gently whisper the circle back in ways that are 'old and new'?

To me, these three communities show that a more healing

way is possible. In them, I see hope. Not the hope that needs to escape from the here and now but the hope of knowing a more healing way of living is already being lived by dissimilar people around the world. The power of these stories of healing justice is that they can help us to do the work of reconciliation: awakening us from slumber, helping us to see ourselves in this huge mess, and gently whispering the circle back.

My impression has been that the area of greatest overlap is not common processes or practices but a shared imagination. I have identified six basic wisdoms of healing justice.

Wisdom of Land and Spirit

Healing justice does not begin with states and institutions. Healing justice, as practiced by these communities, begins and ends with the Spirit and the land. For each of these communities, healing justice came from a journey into old wisdom teachings. They trace this justice to the heart of and gift from the Creator. Each community had a different name and understanding of this spirit. However, all communities argue that, if one wants to create and sustain a healing kind of justice, one needs to be in a particular relationship with Spirit and land.

Both Spirit and land push a sense of justice beyond the individual orientation and beyond the state orientation. In fact, this kind of justice is not primarily about social control but more about cultivating a life that acknowledges and responds to the gift, beauty, and fragility of life.

When the land becomes a teacher of justice, the goal is to find wholeness by finding a common connection. The goal of justice is more to (re) discover a sustainable and good balance in the local community than it is to impose a hierarchical state order on distant lands.

Wisdom of Transforming Patterns

When one begins with a broad view of justice, as something sacred, as something reflected in the wisdom of the Earth that involves balance, harmony, and wholeness, then it follows that the procedures of justice involve transforming relationships and patterns within the whole system. This does not follow the typical wisdom of rules and procedures. Here, justice is a creative act of staying close to those who suffer as they demonstrate, like canaries in a mine, those aspects of the environment that lead to harm rather than healing. The wisdom of transforming patterns is one that seeks to understand the root causes and conditions of harm and to break the unhealthy patterns that lead to such harm. It intimately links the episode of harm to the structures, patterns, and relationships that encourage such harm. This wisdom expands the horizon of time and widens the relevant who. When the horizon of time expands, then we stop dealing with Meer incidents, and rather seek patterns, generations, and structures. Rather than primarily blaming individuals, it responds to harm as an opportunity to transform the whole community.

Wisdom of Cultivating the Conditions of Loving-Kindness

Rather than a kind of justice rooted in responding to harms (the wisdom of problem responsiveness), healing justice is rooted in the wisdom of cultivating the conditions of loving-kindness. This wisdom of justice does not wait for harm or symptomatic episodes. It seeks to cultivate the conditions for loving-kindness. This wisdom sees healing justice as an exploration of the kind of social, economic, and political conditions that do not lead to harm but loving-kindness. This wisdom is interested in how to organize a community in such a way as to lead to joy. When harm happens, this wisdom does not focus all its attention on the negative. It believes that demonstrating loving-kindness is the way of awakening those who have forgotten how to act in such a way. The wisdom of cultivating the conditions of loving-kindness then has a double goal: to avoid the environments that cause harm while cultivating the environments that lead to the fullness of life.

Wisdom of Finding True Identity

Rather than labeling victims, offenders, and professional helpers, healing justice seeks to reveal to each person their true names. Inspired by watching land and Spirit, one's true names are about how we are connected to 'others.' Those who have forgotten how to act as good relatives need to be reminded of what it is to be a good relation. Those who suffer harm are often seen as one who is out of balance – in danger of forgetting their essential natures, their true names. The wisdom of finding true names means justice must create space to explore, identify, and to rediscover how all things are connected. This wisdom does not try to create good by telling people they are essentially bad. Rather, it tries to awaken the compassion for the other by teaching about one's true nature and the nature of our mutual interdependence. This wisdom assumes that those who live in forgetfulness of these things need to be surrounded by a caring community that will help them remember who they are. These communities do not have a single universal process, as this kind of wisdom seeks to understand identity both in its particularity and interconnectedness.

Wisdom of Interdependent Relationships

Healing justice is not wisdom that turns on individual autonomy. It is a wisdom of interdependent relationships. Because all things are seen as essentially interconnected, responsibility and accountability are understood communally. Rather than blaming the individuals, this wisdom moves to understand how families, villages, and countries raise the kind of people who harm others. At the same time, this wisdom focuses on transforming those same sets of relationships to cultivate healing justice. This wisdom of interdependent relationships is different from the wisdom of states. This wisdom gives preference to locally-based and locally driven harms responses over state-based and state-driven ones. It is interested in transforming the whole collective – in its memory, its structures, its relationships, and its patterns of behavior. This wisdom of interdependent relationships sees healing justice as creating community – creating social, economic, and political structures – rooted in a healing perspective.

Wisdom of Healing for All

This wisdom sees healing as the interpretative framework for justice. Rather than punishment, it sees healing as both the means and ends of justice. While healing justice is not always a justice free of punishment, punishment does not become the central interpretative framework. Healing justice is rooted in a justice that respects the sacredness of each person and believes that all can heal. This wisdom of healing then does not rely so heavily on punishment and violence as a last resort. This wisdom sees the world as constantly changing, open both to changing towards healing and changing towards harm. The wisdom of healing for all sees harms as an opportunity to work at healing for all involved – the ones harmed and the ones harming. It also works to transform the family, the socio-economic and ecological structures.

The wisdom of healing for all returns us to the wisdom of Spirit and land, in whom all find their true identity.

Final Words

In comparing these stories, I discovered there was a broad basis of similarity between them. Healing justice, at least as found in these three communities, has commonalities in vision, is practiced through strategies that have similarities, and is critically dependent on certain kinds of relationships and structures. We can say with confidence that healing justice exists even in the modern world.

The communities in this book have been my teachers helping me to see a new horizon of justice. I thank them for opening up different ways of seeing and being, and I acknowledge that I am yet a toddler, barely learning to walk in the ways of healing justice.

The reader should not be misled. Healing justice comes from senses of beauty, compassion, and deep peace. Some might find this appealing. However, healing justice gains its power by entering the painful sufferings of the world. It is not an easy path. It does not come simply. The communities and people I met were not perfect. They struggled as the way forward that had seemed so promising became obscured.

THEY WERE ALSO JOYFUL, but their joy did not come from trying to escape suffering. Their joy came from knowing they could stand in the midst of suffering and not be ashamed, fearful, or vengeful. The more they learned to see with the eyes of compassion, the more they understood the depths of suffering. Healing justice leads to joy in the midst of suffering.

THOSE WHO EXPECT justice to control suffering and to deal with suffering so that they do not have to would do well to stay far away from healing justice. It will surely disappoint.

Those who wish to pursue healing justice are invited to do so in ways that embody healing justice. There is more that we do not understand about healing justice than what we do understand. More research is needed but, even more important than research, more demonstration plots of healing justice are needed for us to understand it better.

This book shares stories of communities living a healing justice. Healing justice is not something fixed that we can hold onto and control. It is more of a wise imagination for how to live in the world. Healing justice comes as gift. It disappears or recedes when not treated as such. I believe these stories have great implication for those with the capacity to listen. I hope this book dares readers to find their own way to practice healing justice.

Please Leave a Star Rating

Enjoy This Book? You Can Make a Big Difference

Ratings are the most powerful tool when it comes to getting attention for my books. The secret to getting my books noticed is:

A committed and loyal bunch of readers like you.

Honest ratings of my books help bring them to the attention of other readers.

If you enjoyed this book, I would be very grateful if you could spend five minutes leaving a rating on Amazon. If you wish, you can leave an honest review also. These can be as short as a few words.

To leave a rating, use one of the links below.

- https://www.amazon.com/review/create-review/ref=dpx_acr_wr_link?asin=B07G67TC9P#
- https://www.amazon.ca/review/create-review/ref=dpx_acr_wr_link?asin=B07G67TC9P• *https://www.amazon.com/dp/B07G67TC9P*
- https://www.amazon.co.uk/review/create-review/ref=acr_dpproductdetail_solicit?ie=UTF8&asin=B07G67TC9P
- https://www.goodreads.com/book/show/41014247-healing-justice

Acknowledgments

All story-telling is, of course, communal. In telling stories, we enter a web of relationships, and even our observing changes their nature and our nature. What we see is not just dependent on what is there. We see through the lens molded by those who have gone before us. We cannot help but stand on the shoulders of our ancestors, our mentors, and our enemies. Each shapes what we see, how we see it, and what meaning we attach to it. As I have learned from the communities in this study, acknowledging the gifts of those who have gone before is an important part of doing healing justice.

At the heart of this book are three wonderful communities. While each had grounds to be suspicious of academic university research, each agreed to participate in the research and to host me as I tried to learn as much as I could about their approaches to healing justice. I would like to thank the Elders and community of Hollow Water, Manitoba, Canada for agreeing to participate in this research. In particular, I would like to thank Burma Bushie, Marcel Hardisty, Sharon Klyne, Jeanette Cook, Randy Ducharme, Gabriel Hall, Bernie Hardisty, Laura Hardisty, Marilyn Sinclair, Donna Smith and the rest of the staff at Circle Healing and Community Holistic Program. In Plum Village, I would like to thank Thich Nhat Hanh, Sister Chân Không, Pháp Liêu, Chân Tùng Nghiêm, Đào Nghiêm, Dinh Nghiêm, Mai Nghiêm, Nhủ Nghiêm, Tôn Nghiêm, Trish Thompson, Pháp Xả and the rest of the monks and nuns at Plum Village in France. In the Iona Community in Scotland (and beyond), I would like to thank Kathy Galloway, Graeme Brown, Ruth Burgess, Tom Gordon, Desirée van der Hijden, Nick Prance, Zam Walker, Richard Sharples and Biddy Sharples. It is a deep honour to enter the imagination, stories, traumas, and joys of another person and other communities. It is also a great responsibility. I have tried from the beginning to end to conduct this research in respectful ways. I deeply thank these communities for sharing their ways, for being my teachers, and for encouraging me to practice the habits of healing justice within the concrete fabric of my life.

I would like to thank my colleagues at Canadian Mennonite University for supporting me and providing a home base. I thank Jessica Kingsley Publisher for returning to me my rights to these stories.

A number of colleagues have made important contributions to this work by reading and critiquing parts of this manuscript. I would like to thank Howard Zehr, Rupert Ross, Tom Fisher, Len Sawatsky, and Michael Bischoff. A special thank you goes to Gerry Johnstone and Tony Ward, who met with me regularly and provided invaluable input and encouragement throughout this research.

A number of people also helped with the editing of this work. Thank you to Rhona Sawatsky, Roger Gateson, and especially to Albert Labun, who with great care, attention, and love worked with me at each stage.

I especially thank my family, my mother, Donelle Sawatsky, who demanded that I study the law of love and who died during this research, and my father, Len Sawatsky, who introduced me to restorative justice while I was still a child. I would express my gratitude to our friends at Grain of Wheat Church Community. And finally, my family – to Rhona, Sara, and Koila – who accompanied me in so many ways in this journey into healing justice. I thank you.

Resources and References

On Plum Village

Cao, N. P. (1993). *Learning true love: how I learned and practiced social change in Vietnam*. Berkeley: Parallax Press.

Hanh, T. N. (1967). *Vietnam: lotus in a sea of fire*. New York: Hill and Wang.

Hanh, T. N. (1987a). *Being peace*. Berkeley, Calif.: Parallax Press.

Hanh, T. N. (1987b). *The sutra on the eight realizations of the Great Beings: A Buddhist scripture on simplicity, generosity, and compassion*. Berkeley, Calif.: Parallax Press.

Hanh, T. N. (1991). *Peace is every step: the path of*

459

mindfulness in everyday life. New York, N.Y.: Bantam Books.

Hanh, T. N. (1992a). *Breathe! You are alive: sutra on the full awareness of breathing*. London: Rider.

Hanh, T. N. (1992b). *Touching peace: practicing the art of mindful living*. Berkeley, Calif.: Parallax Press.

Hanh, T. N. (1993). *Call me by my true names: the collected poems of Thich Nhat Hanh*. Berkeley, Calif.: Parallax Press.

Hanh, T. N. (1995). *Zen keys: a guide to Zen practice*. London: Thorsons.

Hanh, T. N. (1998). *Fragrant palm leaves: journals, 1962-1966*. Berkeley, Calif.: Parallax Press.

Hanh, T. N. (2001). *Anger: wisdom for cooling the flames*. New York: Riverhead Books.

Hanh, T. N. (2002a). *Be free where you are*. Berkeley, Calif.: Parallax Press.

Hanh, T. N. (2002b). 'Go as a Sangha.' In T. N. Hanh and J. Lawlor (eds) *Friends on the path* Berekley: Parallex Press: 17-48.

Hanh, T. N. (2002c). 'Spirituality in the twenty-first century.' In T. N. Hanh and J. Lawlor (eds) *Friends on the path* Berkeley: Parallax Press: 9-16.

Hanh, T. N. (2003a). 'Compassion is our hope: practicing to reduce violence in society'. *Protecting and serving without stress or fear*, Green Lake, WI: Plum Village Productions.

Hanh, T. N. (2003b). *Finding our true home : living in the Pure Land here and now*. Berkeley, Calif.: Parallax Press.

Hanh, T. N. (2003c). *I have arrived, I am home: celebrating twenty years of Plum Village life*. Berkeley, Calif.: Parallax.

Hanh, T. N. (2003d). 'I have arrived, I am home: dharma talk '. *Protecting and serving without stress or fear*, Green Lake, Wisconsin: Plum Village Productions.

Hanh, T. N. (2003e). *Joyfully together: the art of building a harmonious community*. Berkeley, Calif.: Parallax Press.

Hanh, T. N. (2003f). 'Mindfulness of anger: embracing the child within'. *Protecting and serving without stress or fear*, Green Lake, WI: Plum Village Productions.

Hanh, T. N. (2003g). 'Right thinking: the code of law'. *Protecting and serving without stress or fear*, Green Lake, WI: Plum Village Productions.

Hanh, T. N. (2005). 'Creating our environment: building a foundation of stability and peace'. *Colors of compassion 2005: healing our families, building true community*, Escondido, CA: Plum Village Productions.

Hanh, T. N. (2007). *For a future to be possible: Buddhist ethics for everyday life*. Berkeley, CA: Parallax Press.

Hanh, T. N. and J. Lawlor (2002). *Friends on the path: living spiritual communities*. Berkeley, Calif.: Parallax.

Hanh, T. N. and Monks and Nuns at Plum Village (2007). *Chanting from the heart: Buddhist ceremonies and daily practices*. Berkeley, Calif.: Parallax Press.

Loy, D. (2001). 'Healing justice: a Buddhist perspective.' In M. L. Hadley (eds) *The spiritual roots of restorative justice* Albany University of New York Press: 81-97.

Monks and Nuns at Plum Village (2003). *How to enjoy your stay in Plum Village: an introduction to Plum Village* Berkeley, Calif: Parallax Press.

Plum Village delegation (2006). 'Buddhism responding to the needs of the 21st century'. *World Buddhist Forum*, Hangzhou, China: http://www.plumvillage.org/general/Buddhism%20Responding%20to%20the%20Needs%20of%20the%2021st%20Century.pdf.

On Hollow Water Community

Bopp, J., M. Bopp, et al. (2002). *Mapping the healing journey: the final report of a First Nation research project on healing in Canadian Aboriginal communities*. Ottawa, Solicitor General Canada: 1-93.

Bushie, B. (1997a). 'CHCH reflections: Burma.' (eds) *Four circles of Hollow Water* Ottawa: Solicitor General Canada Aboriginal Corrections Policy Unit.

Bushie, B. (1997b). 'Hollow Water circle: a personal

reflection.' (eds) *Four circles of Hollow Water* Ottawa: Solicitor General Canada Aboriginal Corrections Policy Unit.

Bushie, B. (1997c). 'W'daeb-awae': the truth as we know it.' (eds) *Four circles of Hollow Water* Ottawa: Solicitor General Canada Aboriginal Corrections Policy Unit.

Bushie, B. (1999). 'Community holistic circle healing: a community approach'. *Building Strong Partnerships for Restorative Practices Conference*, Burlington, Vermont.

Bushie, J. (1997d). 'CHCH reflections: Joyce.' (eds) *Four circles of Hollow Water* Ottawa: Solicitor General Canada Aboriginal Corrections Policy Unit.

Community Holistic Circle Healing Hollow Water (1996). 'Hollow Water First Nation position on incarceration ' In C. C. o. J. a. C. (Canada) (eds) *Satisfying justice: safe community options that attempt to repair harm from crime and reduce the use or length of imprisonment* Ottawa: Church Council on Justice and Corrections (Canada): XXII-XXV.

Couture, J. (2001a). 'Comments on Hollow Water community healing'. *Mental health of Indigenous Peoples*, Montreal: McGill University.

Couture, J. (2001b). *A cost-benefit analysis of Hollow Water's Community Holistic Circle Healing process.* Ottawa: Solicitor General Canada.

Dickie, B. and J. MacDonald (2000). *Hollow Water*. Montreal, National Film Board of Canada.

Dickson-Gilmore, E. J. and C. La Prairie (2005). *Will the circle be unbroken?: aboriginal communities, restorative justice, and the challenges of conflict and change.* Toronto: University of Toronto Press.

Four Directions International (2001). *Mapping the healing experience of Canadian Aboriginal communities: site visit report for Hollow Water Community Holistic Circle Healing Process.* Cochrane, Four Directions International: 1-20.

Hollow Water Community Holistic Circle Healing (1995). 'The Sentencing Circle: seeds of a community healing process.' *Justice as Healing* Winter.

Lajeunesse, T. (1993). *Community Holistic Circle Healing : Hollow Water First Nation.* [Ottawa, Ont.]: Corrections Branch, Solicitor General Canada, Ministry Secretariat.

Lajeunesse, T. (1996). *Evaluation of the Hollow Water Community Holistic Circle Healing Project.* Ottawa, Solicitor General Canada.

McCaslin, W. D. (2005c). *Justice as healing: Indigenous ways.* St. Paul: Living Justice Press.

National Film Board of Canada (2000). *Hollow Water*. Montréal, Québec, National Film Board of Canada.

Ross, R. (1992). *Dancing with a ghost: exploring Indian reality*. Markham, ON: Octopus Books.

Ross, R. (1995). 'Aboriginal community healing in action: the Hollow Water approach.' *Justice as Healing* Spring.

Ross, R. (1996). *Returning to the teachings: exploring aboriginal justice*. Toronto: Penguin Books.

On The Iona Community

Bell, J. L. and G. Maule (1986). *A touching place: songs for worship from the Iona Community*. Glasgow: Wild Goose Publications.

Burgess, R. (2000a). 'The ministry of healing in the life and worship of the Church.' In R. Burgess and K. Galloway (eds) *Praying for the dawn* Glasgow: Wild Goose Publications: 111-134.

Burgess, R. (2000b). 'Weeping for cities and working for justice.' In R. Burgess and K. Galloway (eds) *Praying for the Dawn* Glasgow: Wild Goose Publications: 37-39.

Burgess, R. and K. Galloway (2000). *Praying for the dawn: a resource book for the ministry of healing*. Glasgow: Wild Goose Publications.

Ferguson, R. (1998). *Chasing the wild goose: the story of the Iona Community*. Glasgow: Wild Goose Publications.

Galloway, K. (2000). 'Justice as healing.' In R. Burgess and K. Galloway (eds) *Praying for the dawn: a resource book for the ministry of healing* Glasgow: Wild Goose Publications: 40-43.

Galloway, K. (2004). *The dream of learning our true name*. Glasgow: Wild Goose.

Gorringe, T. (1996). *God's just vengeance: crime, violence, and the rhetoric of salvation*. Cambridge ; New York: Cambridge University Press.

Gorringe, T. (2002). *A theology of the built environment : justice, empowerment, redemption*. Cambridge: Cambridge University Press.

Macdonald, L. O. (1999). *In good company: women in the ministry*. Glasgow: Wild Goose Publications.

Macleod, G. F. B. M. o. F. (1955). *The place of healing in the ministry of the church*. Glasgow: Iona Community.

Meaden, B. (1999). *Protest for peace*. Glasgow: Wild Goose Publications.

Monteith, W. G. (2000). 'Service of prayers for healing of the Iona Community: a historical and theological perspective.' In R. Burgess and K. Galloway (eds) *Praying for the dawn: a resource book of the ministry of healing* Glasgow: Wild Goose Publications: 17-22.

Morrow, D. (2000). 'Where there is injury... hope for healing in Northern Ireland.' In R. Burgess and K. Galloway (eds) *Praying for the dawn* Glasgow: Wild Goose Publications: 55-58.

Morton, T. R. (1957). *The Iona Community story*. London: Lutterworth Press.

Newell, J. P. (2002). *Each day and each night: Celtic prayers from Iona*. Glasgow: Wild Goose Publications, 2003.

Paynter, N. (2006). *Growing hope: daily readings*. Glasgow: Wild Goose Publishing.

The Iona Community (1991). *The Iona Community worship book*. Glasgow: Wild Goose Publications.

The Iona Community (1996). *What is the Iona Community?*: Wild Goose Publications.

The Iona Community (2001a). *Iona Abbey worship book*. Glasgow: Wild Goose Publications.

The Iona Community (2001b). *The Iona Community: today's challenge, tomorrow's hope*. Glasgow, Wild Good Publications.

The Iona Community (2006). *The Iona Community (brochure)*. Glasgow, Wild Goose Publications.

The Iona Community (2007). *Members 2007 (booklet)*. Glasgow, Wild Goose Publications.

The Iona Community. (n.d.-a). *About the community*. Accessed on 4 April, 2007, at http://www.iona.org.uk/.

The Iona Community. (n.d.-b). *Iona Youth*. Accessed on 4 April, 2007, at http://www.iona.org.uk/.

The Iona Community. (n.d.-c). *Our Worship.* Accessed on June 30th, 2008, at http://www.iona.org.uk/.

The Iona Community. (n.d.-d). *The Rule of the Iona Community.* Accessed on 4 April, 2007, at http://www. iona.org.uk/.

Poems

Rashani. (1991). *The Unbroken.* Used with permission.

Tabobondung, R. (2002). 'Reconciliation.' In J. Bird, L. Land, M. Macadam and D. Engelstad (eds) *Nation to Nation: Aboriginal sovereignty and the future of Canada* Toronto: Irwin Publishing: 1. Used with permission.

Jarem's Website:

www.jaremsawatsky.com

To Rhona, Sara, and Koila
For your teaching, patience, and partnership
on this journey into healing justice
and for the many journeys to come.

About the Author

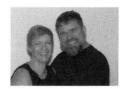

Jarem Sawatsky, Ph.D., is the National Bestselling author/ co-author of 6 books, including the award-winning ***Dancing with Elephants***. He is internationally known for his work as peacebuilder and teacher, working to bring an engaged mindfulness to those interested in wellness, resilience, and transformation. He is Professor Emeritus of Peace and Conflict Transformation Studies at Canadian Mennonite University.

Since being diagnosed with a terminal disease, he has been stumbling his way (literally) into finding more healing and joyful ways to live. He sometimes shares about this journey on his blog. (www.jaremsawatsky. com/dancing-blog).

He lives in Winnipeg, Canada with his wife, twin daughters, and a golden Labrador.

He can be contacted in the following ways:

Website: www.jaremsawatsky.com

Readers Group:

www.jaremsawatsky.com/readers

Made in the USA
Columbia, SC
26 May 2020